NATIONAL INST
SERVICES I

Volume 34

CLAIMANT OR CLIENT?

CLAIMANT OR CLIENT?

A Social Worker's View of the Supplementary Benefits Commission

OLIVE STEVENSON

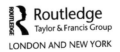

Routledge
Taylor & Francis Group

LONDON AND NEW YORK

First published in 1973 by George Allen & Unwin Ltd

This edition first published in 2022
by Routledge
4 Park Square, Milton Park, Abingdon, Oxon OX14 4RN
605 Third Avenue, New York, NY 10017

Routledge is an imprint of the Taylor & Francis Group, an informa business

British Library Cataloguing in Publication Data
A catalogue record for this book is available from the British Library

ISBN: 978-1-03-203381-5 (Set)
ISBN: 978-1-00-321681-0 (Set) (ebk)
ISBN: 978-1-03-205781-1 (Volume 34) (hbk)
ISBN: 978-1-03-205801-6 (Volume 34) (pbk)
ISBN: 978-1-00-319922-9 (Volume 34) (ebk)

DOI: 10.4324/9781003199229

Publisher's Note
The publisher has gone to great lengths to ensure the quality of this reprint but points out that some imperfections in the original copies may be apparent.

Disclaimer
The publisher has made every effort to trace copyright holders and would welcome correspondence from those they have been unable to trace.

CLAIMANT OR CLIENT?

A SOCIAL WORKER'S VIEW OF
THE SUPPLEMENTARY BENEFITS COMMISSION

OLIVE STEVENSON

London

GEORGE ALLEN & UNWIN LTD

RUSKIN HOUSE   MUSEUM STREET

Printed in Great Britain
in 11 point Fournier type
by Unwin Brothers Limited
Old Woking, Surrey.

ACKNOWLEDGEMENTS

Civil servants traditionally get brickbats rather than bouquets. It is, therefore, a pleasure to record my gratitude to those in the Supplementary Benefits Commission who read this book in detail and offered constructive comments on it. In these, they distinguished at all times between corrections of fact and suggestions about my opinions. I am also deeply appreciative of the speed with which the draft was circulated: it reached the Supplementary Benefits Commission in mid-November and came back to me with comments before Christmas. Lists of names are dull and invidious, and many persons were involved. However, it is appropriate to single out Antony Crocker who rapidly collated his own and others' views and presented them to me with kindness and diplomacy, and Peter Harmston whose advice on the voluntary unemployment chapters was invaluable. Of course others outside the civil service, to whom I am also grateful, have helped me clarify my mind, especially Professor Titmuss. Colleagues in this Department have been much involved, directly and indirectly, and my thanks are particularly due to Michael Hill for the stimulus of his wide knowledge of the subject, to the social work tutors who have been generous about the time the book has taken and to the secretaries who have responded so well to pleas for speed.

Although all case examples used in this book are based on fact, anonymity has been preserved not only through change of name but alterations of details not relevant to the illustration.

O. S.

(Department of Social and Administrative Studies,
The University of Oxford).

INTRODUCTION

The focus of this book has its dangers. It derives from the study made by the writer between 1968 and 1970 of the British Supplementary Benefits Commission. In analysing the strengths and weaknesses of the present system it does not attempt, except in passing references, to make comparisons with similar institutions in other countries or to draw attention to the many parallels in other sectors of the social services. Unfortunately, therefore, the book may encourage those scapegoating processes it was intended to correct since it will not show how our provisions compare with others or how universal some of the problems are to all aspects of our social services. The writer's hope, however, is that it will encourage a more reflective consideration of the fundamental issues involved in the admission of a means-tested benefit scheme which is, in effect, 'the safety net' of our social security scheme.

Readers will note two major omissions. The first is that Reception Centres, an important aspect of the work of the Supplementary Benefits Commission are not discussed. The second is that the place of the Appeal Tribunal in the total structure is not adequately considered. These omissions should not be taken to mean that the writer does not consider them to be of major significance. The explanation is simple. It was not possible in a period of eighteen months as Social Work Adviser to study every aspect of the Commission's work. Indeed, there was a grave danger of superficiality in what was attempted. As to Reception Centres, their work merits much closer examination; provision for 'homeless single persons' is a vital aspect of our social services. Appeal Tribunals are crucial to the credibility of the scheme as a whole, since they involve (potentially) all claimants. But the writer preferred not to embark on discussion of areas of which she did not have first hand experience as Social Work Adviser.

This book has been written from a social worker's viewpoint. It should not be thought, however, that this emphasis implies a complacent view of social workers' present skills and their contribution to the amelioration of social distress. There is certainly no intention of conveying that injections of social work skills into the Supplementary Benefits system would work miracles. It may well be that there are deficiencies or intractable disadvantages in the present structure that only radical change of law or of organisation would remedy. Furthermore, social workers are, or should be, aware of the criticisms that have been levelled at them: first, of inadequate evaluation of the skills they have practised with emotional conviction; second, of reactionary tendencies in working to paper over the cracks of an unsatisfactory social structure. The worker is aware that this last accusation may be levelled at much of this book. The justification is twofold: it is agreed even by its most stringent critics that the British Supplementary Benefits scheme is one of the best of its kind in the world; and the writer is, temperamentally and by training, inclined to work for change rather than revolution. Nothing the writer saw as Social Work Adviser to the Supplementary Benefits Commission convinced her that its present workings were, in general, incompatible with the values of a civilised and human society, with the possible exception of the co-habitation rule. This is not to deny the many deficiencies of the scheme in its present operation—deficiencies with which much of this book will be concerned. It does, however, suggest that moderate improvements, if they are continuous and initiated soon, may avert a head-on collision between social security and social work, which some fear and some foster.

CHAPTER 1

STIGMA AND NEED

Recent History

The history of the Poor Law is familiar ground to any student of the social services and has been excellently documented. Its significance for the discussion that follows is considerable. It is impossible to understand events leading up to and following the passing of the National Assistance Act in 1948 without a historical perspective.

The National Assistance Board did not spring into life fully grown in 1948. The Unemployment Assistance Board came into being in the 1930s when the cover provided by the Unemployment Insurance Scheme with respect to prolonged unemployment was firmly defined and responsibility for those whose insurance benefit was exhausted was transferred from local authority public assistance to a national authority. During the war the supplementary pensions scheme was introduced under the same authority as an alternative to raising the rates of contributory pensions. Thus, when the National Assistance Bill came before Parliament, central government machinery for the relief of need was already established.

The Bill, transferring responsibility for means-tested relief of need from the local authorities to central government, was the last of the new famous social measures of the post-war government to be brought before the House. To read the debates[1] is at once moving and saddening. Seldom can a measure of such importance have provoked so little controversy—a fact remarked upon by some Members. The reasons for this are not hard to trace. A kind of euphoria, natural in a post-war situation, was evident in the political mood of the time; this was by no means unrealistic in terms of the remarkable achievements of the social legislation in this period. To this must be added the hatred—a word not too strong—of the governing party for the old Poor Law. Many Members had had first-hand experience of the indignities and humiliations inherent in the old system. Indeed, it may not be far-fetched to suggest that for some the origins of their

---

[1] For the debates from which the subsequent extracts are taken, see Hansard, Vol. 444, November 1947.

socialist philosophy may have been rooted in such experiences, especially in childhood. Even allowing for the conventions of political overstatement, the debates leave one in no doubt about the passionate sincerity with which the Bill was welcomed. The late Mrs Braddock as always lent colour to the debate but her sentiments were echoed by others.

'There are thousands of people in this country who will welcome this Bill . . . Let us remember the queues outside the Public Relief offices . . . lining up for their weeks ration of black treacle and bread. Bread was issued once a week . . . I have been in a committee where the chairman persisted—and I protested—in seeing the under-clothing of old people before the Committee was prepared to give an order that new underclothing should be supplied. *These things remain with us. We remember them*' (My italics).

Tory politicians were, understandably, less intense in their feelings, but the guilt and the shame of past treatment of the poor hung over the debate, a point taken by Mr Tom Brown who commented: 'I have been trying to discover the cause of the placid atmosphere . . . I think it must be the weight of shame that has been resting upon us.' Few voices were raised, such as would undoubtedly be heard now, on the possibilities of the exploitation of the scheme or on the diffi-culties that might arise in its implementation. One Member struck a conventional note of warning, albeit couched in somewhat colourful terms: 'We should not attempt . . . to encourage people to behave as adult babies, anxious to make use of the public feeding bottle.'

But for the most part the debate was on the side of the poor. The then Secretary of State for Scotland (Rt. Hon. Arthur Woodburn) summed up the Government view: 'We establish in this Bill one of the greatest slogans or ambitions in the early days of our movement—the establishment of work or maintenance . . . as the moral principle governing the treatment of people who are in need . . . Under this measure those who get assistance get it without humiliation or abuse . . . The destruction of the dignity of man was the greatest crime against the poor in days gone by.' This intense emotionalism, com-pounded of post-war optimism and guilt for past sins against the poor, did not make for constructive debate. One of the few serious warnings came from Mr Albert Evans, Member for Islington West: 'If . . . stigma is to go, it will need something more than this Bill, or an Act . . . or Regulations. [The administrators] . . . have to humanise the relation-ships between the poor and authority.' This statement is in interesting contrast to that of the then Minister of Health (Aneurin Bevan) who, introducing the Bill, said:

'[The Government] wish to consider assistance by way of monetary help made a national responsibility and welfare a local responsibility. Where the individual is immediately concerned, where warmth and humanity of administration is the primary consideration, then the authority which is responsible should be as near to the recipient as possible.'

The assumptions in this statement are twofold: first, that the administration of monetary assistance does not require the 'warmth and humanity' necessary for the administration of other social services; second, that the division of services into 'national' and 'local' is related to the degree of personal contact the individual needs from the services. It is with these issues, among others, that much of this book is concerned.

The changes thus described by Bevan were taken a stage further in 1966 when the National Assistance Board, becoming the Supplementary Benefits Commission, joined with the former Ministry of Pensions and National Insurance to become the Ministry of Social Security. The implications of this will be discussed more fully later. It is sufficient to note that the amalgamation marked a further consolidation of income maintenance services within a centralised system.

However, before considering the workings of the Supplementary Benefits scheme within the framework of social security, three issues which are of central importance to the theme of this book must be discussed. The first of these concerns the stigma attached to means-tested benefits; the second concerns the relation of monetary assistance to other forms of social service; and the third concerns the exercise of discretion in monetary assistance.

The Stigma of Claiming Benefit[1]

Stigma has been defined as 'a stain' on one's good name. Sociologists[2] have drawn attention to the processes by which individuals or groups are stigmatised and the effects on the persons involved. It is clear that such moral opprobrium is frequently associated with poverty, an opprobrium which politicians, social reformers and social workers

---

[1] I am indebted to Professor Titmuss for help on clarifying this issue.
[2] See, for example, E. Goffman, *Stigma: Notes on the Management of Spoiled Identity,* Prentice Hall, New Jersey, 1963.

have increasingly sought to eliminate but which is associated with the sense of failure in a materialistic culture.

However, problems of stigmatisation involve many different people in society and 'the poor' are but one of a number of overlapping groups who may experience it in their relationship to the society in which they live. The processes involved are complex. We have to consider the interaction between those who stigmatise and those who are stigmatised. There are a wide variety of criteria for success in our society of which sexual marital and child-rearing achievements are the most obvious in family life. It happens that, by virtue of its function the Supplementary Benefits Commission brings together in one place—the local office—a number of people whose sense of failure derives not only from poverty but from other failures to achieve the normal 'goods' in society. Thus the unemployed, the handicapped, the separated wife and the mother of an illegitimate child queue together for money. Each in his or her own way feels the guilt and anger associated with failure in a role deemed to be of significance in our society. It can readily be seen, therefore, that the SBC is likely to be the focal point of emotion, not all of which is to do with the stigma of poverty alone.

Perhaps because it has been easier to grapple with, much effort has been directed at reducing the sense of stigma experienced by the elderly in making claims for means-tested benefits and it is clear that this has had considerable success. In the ten years between 1960 and 1970 there was an increase of nearly a million in the number of elderly people receiving supplementary pensions, not all of which can be accounted for by a proportional growth in that sector of the population or an increase in the real value of benefits. It would generally be conceded that in public statements and in the day-to-day treatment of elderly claimants, the NAB and then the SBC have made consistent efforts to 'destigmatise' benefit and to bury the ghosts of the past. Yet there remains a profound ambivalence in society, above all in relation to unemployed men and fatherless families, between the idea of stigma-free entitlement to various forms of state benefit on the one hand and of deterrence to avoid exploitation on the other. The latter rests on a genuine doubt concerning the strength of individual motivation towards self-reliance if incentives are weakened. This persistent anxiety about abuse affects the attitudes of those who provide and those who claim and plays a part in maintaining an element of stigma within the system. What is not always appreciated by the general public, however, is the fundamental difference between the provision of positive incentives towards financial independence (such as encouragement of part-time work) and those aspects of an administrative process that tend to reduce the dignity and individuality of the claimant. There is evidence from past experience and from modern sociological studies[1] to support the view that the latter may reinforce that which it is desired to avoid—in this case, exploitative dependence. Indeed, the problem of stigma may be seen in its most tragic form among those who appear to feel it least. For some, continuous experience (and parental experience) of dependent poverty engenders apparent acceptance of a 'failure role' in society. Paradoxically, it may be for these persons that any attack on the stigmatising process is most relevant, rather than for those who are, for example, dismayed or disgusted by their first experience in a local Supplementary Benefits office.

As this book is being written, rising unemployment is causing increasing concern. Should this continue, it will mean that an increasing number of men will be paid supplementary benefit when unemployment benefit is exhausted. It is possible that this will have an impact on the administration of the Supplementary Benefits scheme, comparable in some ways to the effects of large-scale unemployment on the administration of 'outdoor relief' in the 1930s. In a period of full employment, men receiving supplementary benefit (excluding a large group of the elderly whose supplementary pension is, in effect, simply a supplement of their contributory pensions) are, in a sense, stigmatised from the outset as 'failures'. Large-scale unemployment blurs the distinctions and the least adequate in our society can camouflage themselves in the queue alongside the others. This point can be expanded in relation to the Supplementary Benefits claimants generally and indeed to others who live in, or on the margins of, poverty. Increasing general prosperity in which the majority can share highlights the minority who, for a variety of economic, social or psychological reasons, do not share in it. Thus a prosperous society that gives special benefits to 'the poor' is bound to increase the sense of stigma of the few and the noise of their protest is rarely ever more than a whisper. (There has recently been an upsurge of activity on the part of the Claimants' Unions who are often forceful and vociferous in representing the needs of their members but so far only a small number of claimants have been affected.)

Successive governments have hoped to reduce or eliminate stigma

[1] See, for example, E. Goffman, *Asylums*, Anchor Doubleday, New York, 1961; Penguin, Harmondsworth, 1970.

B

in means-tested benefits by changes in the structure and processes of administration. Thus the National Assistance Board would, it was hoped, achieve the miracle by transferring functions from local to central government. The then Parliamentary Secretary to the Ministry of Health expressed this hope in the closing debate on the National Assistance Bill: 'I think it would be difficult to exaggerate the importance of this occasion . . . Poverty is no longer a crime . . . [It was said that] a mere change of administrative form is not itself significant. That may be true of those who live excessively in the realm of cold logic but for the majority of us . . . change in administrative form is significant.'

In 1966, the creation of the Ministry of Social Security was in part justified on the grounds that it would: 'end the sharp distinction we have today . . . for administration of contributory and non-contributory benefits in order to meet the feeling . . . that a non-contributory benefit is inferior in kind and savours of charity' (Miss M. Herbison, then Minister of Pensions and National Insurance).[1]

In this statement the association of stigma with charitable relief is made. Given that some relative poverty is inevitable, the argument runs, we can reduce stigma by a process of depersonalisation. Thus the responsibility for administering benefits was given in 1948 to central government, taking away (it was argued) the danger of local intrusiveness into personal affairs. Then stigma could be further reduced by bringing such non-contributory benefits administratively closer to contributory benefits. That is to say, the notions of right and of eligibility would carry more conviction if the scheme were associated with insurance schemes in which benefits are related to (although far from fully covered by) contributions.

No impartial observer looking at the differences in attitude to the giving and receiving of means-tested benefits between the 1930s and the present day can deny that progress has been made in reducing stigma, both by the major structural changes described above and by a host of administrative improvements. For example, between October and December 1966, following the amalgamation, some 600,000 pensioners claimed for the first time. Clearly the publicity campaign was successful, not simply in informing but in convincing such people of their rights. It is equally clear that the high hopes expressed in the 1940s that the National Assistance would abolish all sense of stigma have not been realised and it seems improbable that the

[1] Second reading of the Ministry of Social Security Bill, May 1966.

subsequent changes will have done so. We have to ask, th
whether any changes or improvements can eradicate the proble,
a society so strongly orientated to materialistic values. Is it n
hypocritical to deny the stigma when at the same time society make
clear that achievement is measured to an extent by the acquisition and
display of wealth? This is, of course, no argument for leaving the
problem unattacked. It does, however, suggest that structural changes
by themselves, let alone political slogans, cannot reassure claimants
that they have nothing to be ashamed of, not only because of the
impact of the Poor Law which one would expect to decrease in time,
but also because of the value society places on effort that has material
objectives. The lack of public comprehension about the basis of
contributory benefits and particularly of the limited extent to which
today's retirement pensioners have paid for their pension by contributions helps not at all and it is at least open to argument that the
abolition of this hypothetical connection between the individual's
'input' and 'output' would go some way to blurring the distinction
that still exists, despite ministerial amalgamations, between contributory and non-contributory benefits. The improbability of this
taking place reflects society's unwillingness to accept fully and un-
equivocally the responsibility of the stronger to support the weaker
or, indeed, to agree a definition of 'weaker', with the possible exception
of the elderly. We cling to the idea of individual insurance against
poverty and related problems thus, by implication, stigmatising those
who have not been able to make such provision and reinforcing the
very attitudes that it is claimed must be eradicated.

Stigma at the Local Level
Thus far, the stigmatising process has been considered in terms of
the larger issues of social policy. However, such considerations may
seem remote and of little significance to the claimants for whom local
conditions and the attitudes of the individuals administering benefit
may be important in convincing them that 'there is no stain on their
good name'.
　　To read Mrs Braddock's account of queuing for bread and treacle
or of showing underwear to a committee to request renewal is to be
reminded of the enormous progress that has been made, in a relatively
short period, in administering benefit with respect for the recipient.
(Benefits 'in kind' are still given in public assistance schemes in the
USA). Basic changes in principles and practices have done much to
reduce the stigma. One of the most striking examples of a change

principle was the abolition of the household means test and the restriction of financial liability for dependents to the immediate family. These two changes did much to reinforce the dignity of the individual in need since they reduced the degree of dependence on others which had in some cases exacerbated family tensions and placed intolerable strain on the unit it was desired to protect. (This situation still exists in some parts of the USA and in Israel, in both of which countries the scheme is administered by social workers.) As to changes in practice, one might perhaps single out as an important example the issue of order books, linked to the expansion of a visiting service: for very many claimants, especially the elderly, visits to local offices thus became unnecessary. Weekly attendances at offices were routine in the days before 1948 and there are officers in the Commission now who can recall the queues of elderly people presenting their paid-up rent books before receiving their weekly allowances.

That there are no grounds for complacency, however, is clear from the criticisms of claimants, social workers and others and from the expressed anxiety of Commission members concerning, for example, poor office conditions and pressures on overworked staff. Criticism of the conditions under which claimants are interviewed in local offices has been widespread. It is obviously an important issue in increasing or diminishing the feeling of stigma. Whether women are more sensitive to this issue, or just more articulate about it, is not clear. Remarks such as the following, made by women, are certainly not uncommon:[1]

'I felt terrible and when I got down there I felt a damn sight worse— so many people there and afraid of somebody coming in and seeing me that I knew. Degrading.'

'It's degrading. I have always been so independent. You get all the scruffs of London in that office.'

'Long waits while you sit and do nothing with things churning round in your head. Waiting and thinking get you in such a state that you know you won't be able to talk properly when its your turn.'

But improved accommodation, however desirable, does not solve all the problems. As had been said, fewer of the elderly call to claim benefit. This means that the 'caller' population consists in the main

[1] These were individual communications from women to Supplementary Benefits Research Officers.

of unemployed men and some women. The latter are usually in a state of domestic crisis, otherwise they would be in receipt of order books. Among the callers there are bound to be a number whose appearance and behaviour mark them out as socially unacceptable to most people in society. In local offices one must expect to see itinerants, alcoholics, drug addicts, prostitutes and so on. It would be naive to suppose that improved office conditions could remove the sense of stigma-by-association that many people feel, especially in view of their own sense of role failure, as discussed earlier. The out-patient department of a hospital similarly represents a cross-section of society and some distaste at one's bench companions may also be felt in that situation. Yet it is not so intense or so common. This serves to illustrate the underlying sense of failure associated with poverty and what led up to it, in contrast to sickness. There is a hypersensitivity to this particular situation.

Among staff, however, there is some dispute about the value claimants place on improved office accommodation. Some can give examples of new offices and new equipment that have remained in good condition after heavy use and that have, in contrast to the old ones, been treated well by claimants. Such experiences suggest that, as with so much else in the social services, notably housing, improved conditions lead to improved behaviour and accord with the social workers' expectation that decent treatment begets decent behaviour. Other officials, however, can cite depressing examples of new premises ruined in a short period—seats slashed, walls defaced, and so on. Such differences in experience lead one to consider the dynamics of the local office situation. It may be that conscientious attempts to improve physical conditions without concurrent attention to the actual processes within an office are likely to fail. For example, the length of waiting time and at what stages in the process the waiting takes place—that is to say, whether it is before a claim is made or after eligibility has been determined—make a considerable difference to the tensions of the individual concerned. Payment by Giro orders is now normal practice. This has drastically reduced waiting time and it is hoped that it will thus reduce tension in the office although there are still some overburdened caller sections. Thus attempts to improve material conditions or local organisation need to be related to the attitudes and feelings of claimants.

This particular situation engenders tension in everyone. The claimant is, in effect, asking for the means of life itself. Feelings are expressed in different ways, some of which are disruptive and distressing to other claimants and some of which are contagious in a group situation, especially when delays occur. This makes the structure and dynamics of local offices a potent force for good or ill with respect to the sense of stigma. This was recognised by the then Minister of Pensions and National Insurance who, in introducing the second reading of the Ministry of Social Security Bill, gave as one reason for the amalgamation of the Ministry of Pensions and National Insurance with the new-styled Supplementary Benefits Commission that there would be 'one comprehensive service for the public, dealing at one point of contact'—a plan aimed at reducing stigma as well as at simplifying the processes for inquiries. Progress in achieving these 'integrated' social security offices has been inevitably and predictably slow and although about 130 offices are now integrated there are still different inquiry points for 'insurance' and supplementary benefits callers, largely because the schemes are too complicated for one receptionist to deal with both. Such reorganisation is therefore of considerable practical complexity. Whether it can achieve one of its desired results—that of blurring the distinction between recipients of contributory and non-contributory benefits—is doubtful.

The Attitudes of Officials

Finally, and of profound importance in this discussion of the problem of stigma, there is the question of the attitudes of officials and of the interaction between officials and claimants. Clearly attitudes of implicit or explicit contempt can do much to exacerbate the problem and it would be naive to suppose that such attitudes were not on occasion apparent. There are many complex factors underlying such feelings. The implied assumption of superiority may spring from a fundamental lack of sympathy for, or interest in, some claimants who frequent local offices. Officials of the SBC may not have chosen this field of work when entering the Civil Service[1] and may find such contacts quite uncongenial. Apparent contempt, however, may derive from thinly veiled insecurity in which superiority is asserted out of a mixture of fear, anxiety and ignorance in face of aggressive or disturbed claimants. It must also be related to a more generalised anxiety between groups in society, in which the new-found and/or hardly-won respectability of the working or lower-middle classes confronts the apparent improvidence or immorality of the claimant. It must be remembered that many of the civil servants who meet the claimants face to face come from these classes in society.

[1] See Chapter 8.

However, it is important that the extent of such attitudes should not be exaggerated. Even where they do exist beneath the surface the standards of civility and courtesy among British civil servants goes a considerable way toward masking them. To the extent that contemptuous attitudes do exist, they are often the product of tensions related to the current dynamics of the office. Social workers, familiar now with a variety of theories of interaction, will not find it difficult to apply these to the local offices of Supplementary Benefits. In this situation, clerical officers (that is to say, officers of low status and relatively low pay in the organisation) are required in office interviews to establish eligibility and to recommend payments for claimants, some of whom must be described as the most inadequate in our society, some of whom are fraudulent, and some of whom are offensive. (This does not, of course, apply to many who are none of these things.) Moreover, they are required to do this on some days of the week (notably Fridays) under conditions of extreme pressure. Sociologists will point to the role tension engendered on both sides in a relationship in which the claimant sees power as vested in the interviewing officer whereas the clerical officer is only too aware of his obligation to justify a recommendation to an Executive Officer behind the scenes. Psychologists will identify a situation of tension in which the claimant's application for money is of profound emotional significance to both parties, mirroring particular individual attitudes rooted in past experiences. Furthermore, the claimant will on many occasions be hypersensitive to innuendoes of contempt.

Important as it may be to detect and check official attitudes that show blatant prejudice, it is ingenuous to suppose that this alone would reassure claimants, given the background to this problem that has been discussed above. 'Affective neutrality', which is the desired norm for a good bureaucrat, provides interesting opportunities for projection. The derogatory term 'faceless bureaucrat' indicates the fear that many people have of just that impersonal style to which civil servants aspire. Certainly, it is easy to read into such behaviour indications of feeling; the complexities of this kind of interaction are such that it would often be impossible to sort out projection from an accurately received unspoken communication. This leads one to consider the degree of extra awareness of such interaction, beyond that which would be expected of civil servants in other situations, that may be needed by officials in the Supplementary Benefits scheme. Such a suggestion—accepted in principle by the Commission and reflected in current training arrangements—is nevertheless in some conflict with what one might describe as the 'classic' bureaucratic stance and with the tendency discussed earlier, evident since 1948, to *depersonalise* the dispensing of means-tested benefits. The attack on stigma was thought to be most likely to succeed by a process of depersonalisation associated with increased emphasis on 'entitlement', on 'benefit as of right' and a decrease in discretionary powers vested in officials. The question of discretion will be discussed in detail later;[1] for the moment it is sufficient to point out that there are dangers in attempting to 'depersonalise' the encounter between officials and claimants if this means that little account is, or should be, taken of the feelings of the individuals concerned. Even if discretion were completely eliminated (which, as will be shown, it is not and should not be), a means-tested benefit involves inquiries into personal affairs, some of which, as in the case of deserted wives or mothers of illegitimate children, involve questions of an especially intimate nature but which in all cases raise feelings of inadequacy and dependency. Failure to recognise this may cause inaccurate information to be obtained and may actually affect the assessment of basic entitlement since such feelings may lead to confusion in the way a claim is made. Apart from this, however, there can be no doubt that the way these reactions are dealt with will have a profound effect on the sense of stigma. It is not suggested that discussion of such feelings in any depth with claimants is possible or appropriate. But there is no doubt that the officials' awareness of and sympathetic response to them will go some way to improving the communication between them and to alleviating in some degree the sense of shame.

The foregoing discussion has been intended to show how complex is the problem of stigma in this field and, consequently, how complex are the remedies, ranging from large-scale political and administrative changes to local arrangements and attitudes of officials on the spot. Furthermore, behind this lie problems of social attitudes, of criteria for social success and failure generally, which affect the encounters between the officials of the SBC and their claimants. It is small wonder that the political euphoria which greeted the two major post-war changes in the administration of the scheme has not been proved justified. Yet a historical perspective, or indeed a comparison with other countries, gives us some reassurance that progress is being made.

[1] See Chapter 2.

The 'Whole Man'—A 'Blasphemous Abstraction'?[1]

The pattern of our present division between welfare services and the Supplementary Benefits administration was laid down in 1948. The National Assistance Act placed upon local authorities a responsibility for development of residential care for the elderly and others in need of care or attention; this, in conjunction with the 1948 Children Act, was the death blow to the work-house as a part of the public assistance scheme. Since 1948 we have seen the development of increasingly sophisticated social services within the local authorities and the rise of social work as a profession to man them. In the NAB and in the SBC the emphasis has been on the development of a financial service which, while not eliminating discretion, has had as its primary objective the establishment of notions of impartial 'entitlement' and whose administration has been governed by the traditional norms and values of the civil service.

There are three aspects of this division of services which, although connected, are quite distinct. Behind them lies an issue of fundamental importance which is the theme of this book. How do the different facets of human need—economic, social and psychological—relate to each other and how should the services set up to meet these needs be related? The three issues, commonly confused in discussion of the Supplementary Benefits scheme, are: first, the distinction between what has been described by the theologian Tillich[2] as 'creative' (or individualised) justice versus 'proportional' (or equitable) justice; secondly, the unit of government, central or local, that administers such schemes; and thirdly, the personnel, civil servants or social workers, who administer the scheme.

Creative and Proportional Justice

The two different elements in justice, 'creative' and 'proportional', are of the greatest significance in understanding the most important issues and problems in the administration of the Supplementary Benefits scheme. Indeed, it is no exaggeration to suggest that this issue is relevant to most aspects of social work and social policy and is one to which social workers have given little conscious attention, although they experience daily the tension resulting from it. 'Creative' justice is concerned with the uniqueness and therefore the differential

[1] From A. Keith-Lucas, *Decisions about people in Need.* University of Carolina Press, 1957.
[2] P. Tillich, *Love, Power and Justice*, Oxford University Press, 1960.

need of individuals; 'proportional' justice with fairness as between individuals in society.

As has been shown, one aspect of the movement to reduce stigma was a concern to establish a principle of 'entitlement' to benefit. The word, which came into use after the formation of the SBC in 1966 but whose implications were already evident in the NAB, carried an implication of 'a right' rather than 'a need', thus shifting somewhat the formal power relation between the official and the claimant. With this, however, went the expectation that entitlement would be precisely defined by legislation, so as to reduce the extent of individual discretion and decision-making by officials in particular cases. That is to say, 'proportional' justice was emphasised. However, as will be discussed in detail later, neither the NAB nor the SBC have eliminated discretionary powers which represent an element of creative justice in the system. It appears to the writer to be unarguable that a means-tested scheme that is, in effect, a safety net into which people fall when other forms of benefit are not available or have been exhausted, must be flexible or it is a contradiction in terms. This flexibility implies a capacity to respond sensitively to a diversity of financial needs, to the unique circumstances of individuals. Burns,[1] writing of social insurance schemes, describes them as 'a social institution dominated by the concept of average rather than individual need'. She continues: 'This characteristic of social insurance limits the extent to which this form of social security can deal with the total problem of family economic insecurity. A program dealing with average conditions and needs will always have to be supplemented by a system of public assistance to provide for emergencies and special needs.' The state, therefore, cannot abdicate its responsibility for a degree of 'creative justice', of response to individual need, in planning its financial social services. This does not, of course, dispose of the knotty problems concerning its extent, its definition and its administration—good or bad—which will be considered later. It does, however, establish a principle of the utmost importance and one which recent trends both in government and in certain pressure groups, here and in the USA, have tended to depreciate. It is somewhat ironic that in the shift from 'eligibility' to 'entitlement' and in the reaction against the degrading procedures by which eligibility was sometimes established, there may be a new kind of injustice, in which the individual finds there is no rule to fit his own case. Examples of this abound in

[1] E. Burns, *The American Social Security System*, Houghton Miffler Company, Boston, 1951.

complex bureaucratised societies. The British Supplementary Benefits scheme has so far avoided its worst excesses but could easily be driven further into this position if its administration came under mounting attack. For bureaucracy tends to protect itself against criticism by further bureaucratisation, as has happened with New York Public Assistnace, in which the 'welfare rights' programme resulted in an itemisation of rights, down to the last toothbrush.

Needless to say, however, the need for equitable distribution of benefit, governed by rules and administered impartially, is also of profound importance. It was the weakness in this aspect of public assistance administration and its consequent disrepute that was a major factor in the decision to transfer responsibility from local to central government. Theoretically there would have been no need to take the administrative function from the local government unit to improve equity, at any rate between different parts of the country. National scales could have been laid down and financial arrangements made between local government and the national Exchequer to share the financial burdens as between one local authority and another. (In practice, however, such financial liaison is complicated and unlikely to work well.) In any case the bad reputation the scheme had acquired, linked no doubt to the complex relationship between central and local government in the United Kingdom, where local authorities guard their independence zealously, made transfer necessary if there was to be a genuine fresh start. Thus a decision was taken in which, as always, elements of social philosophy and practical politics mingled. It was taken at a time when the personal social services in the local authority were rudimentary or non-existent but when their development was in prospect, especially in relation to the care of the elderly and the deprived child. The problems this structural division were to cause were, unsurprisingly, not foreseen, problems arising from the fragmentation of the needs of the 'whole man' —the phrase which has been described by Keith-Lucas as a 'blasphemous abstraction'.

Public Assistance in the USA

To understand the strength of feeling behind Keith-Lucas' statement, one must consider the situation with regard to income maintenance in the USA. Income maintenance is the responsibility of States and local authorities; there is a much greater element of discretion at all levels and the entitlement restricted to certain categories. It is administered by social workers whose development as a profession was earlier than our own. But social work in such agencies has not been prestigious, least of all in public assistance, and the majority of social workers in public assistance were not fully qualified professionally. Voluntary agencies that could select their clients attracted the most highly qualified social workers. The influence of social workers in voluntary agencies was all-pervasive and affected the attitudes of the (largely) untrained workers in public assistance. They did not carry the professional weight to reappraise, in the light of their experience within vastly different settings and in relation to poor people, some of the theories and values propounded by their colleagues in voluntary settings.

Whether from philosophical yearnings or from a need to rationalise the *status quo*, the role of social work in public assistance in the USA was justified on the grounds of the indivisibility of need—material, social and psychological. Such an assumption was unquestioned, for example, in Towle's[1] influential manual for public assistance workers, published in the mid-1940s, and accords with the somewhat global and omnipotent claims for which social work has more recently been attacked. In fact, as a general proposition, the statement is irrefutable. No elaborate argument is needed to demonstrate the folly of social planning which leaves out of account one or other aspect of human need. There are too many examples in our own country, notably in the field of housing, that illustrate the limitations of material provision without attention to social and psychological needs and vice versa. Those who criticise the idea are in the main seeking to redress the balance within social work which, they argue, has placed undue emphasis on the social and, in particular, the psychological at the expense of the material. Further, and most important, they seek to establish the right of an individual to benefit without, to put it bluntly, 'strings attached'. They fear the intrusiveness of the social workers, who may ask questions irrelevent to the material need and who may, in actuality or in the perception of the client, offer assistance in return for certain kinds of 'improvement' in behaviour. There is no doubt that what has been described as 'the psychiatric deluge'[2] that swept American social work in the 1940s played a significant part in all this. It would generally be agreed that psycho-analytic practice took American social work badly off course in relation to its function

---

[1] C. Towle, *Common Human Needs*, National Association of Social Workers, 1945. London, 1962.

[2] K. Woodruffe, *From Charity to Social Work*, Routledge & Kegan Paul, London, 1962.

and objectives. (Its contribution to the understanding of human behaviour was, and will remain, profound.) Such influences filtered into public assistance agencies, affecting workers, many of whom were untrained and professionally insecure and resulted in an inappropriate application of Freudian theory in which practical requests were believed to require examination at a 'deep level' to uncover their underlying significance. Hence the bitterness of the attacks that sprinkle the pages of American social work journals and that have been given detailed expression by Keith-Lucas: 'The recipient may find himself subject to more or less pervasive control of his life as a condition of receiving assistance.'[1] Examples are cited of relief given in kind, not in cash; of 'requirements', as for instance attendance at clinics; of submitting to decisions about one's life; of supervision with an underlying threat whether perceived or actual of withdrawal of assistance if this is not accepted; and of the possibility of additional benefits as 'the price' of good behaviour. Wilson[2] summed up the reaction of anger and resentment, in which the social scientist, often fundamentally out of sympathy with social work, has played an important part: 'The otherwise objective process of dispensing a material subsidy is mixed with and confused by a theoretical commitment to personalised emotional therapy supposedly demanded by the neurotic character of the caseload.'

As in many other aspects of British social work, British attitudes and feelings, especially among social scientists and young social workers, are coloured by some knowledge, directly or indirectly, of the American experience with public assistance. Unfortunately, however, the extrapolations from the American scene are often inappropriate for they do not take into sufficient account the differences between the two countries culturally, and in social policy and social work in particular. It is useful, therefore, to disengage ourselves from the American experience and to take a cool look at the issues involved within our own context.

The Interaction of Needs

The interaction of the different aspects of human need—material, social and psychological—is obvious. Social work is, by definition, concerned with these interactions and this concern gives it its dis-

---

[1] Keith-Lucas, op. cit.
[2] Wilson, 'Public Welfare and the New Frontier', *Social Service Review*, September, 1962.

tinctive character. To concentrate on any one to the exclusion of any
other is to do violence to the person in need and to collude with those
processes of fragmentation that are increasingly recognised as con-
stituting a serious problem in complex urban societies. Recent reaction
against the psycho-analytic orientation of some social work has
pointed up, quite properly, the importance of material need but one
must avoid the oversimplification of implying that clients 'live by
bread alone'. Of course fine-sounding phrases about other kinds of
need can be used as rationalisations to excuse the lack of bread
but that does not alter this commitment of social work to 'the
whole man'. The poor have a right to other problems beside poverty
and to attribute those problems solely to poverty is insulting. Such
a principle certainly does not lead to the conclusion that social
workers should administer means-tested benefits. It is simply to
suggest that the issues are, however, a great deal more complicated
than the proponents of either side have allowed and much of this
book will be taken up with the detailed examination of these
problems.

There can be few who would now dispute that basic entitlement
should be precisely defined, governed by regulations, available to all
in need and, as such, is suitably administered by civil servants. There
could be no return to unlimited discretion, whatever theory of control
it was related to, whether old style deterrence or new style 'con-
ditioning'. The problem lies in the extent to which such an emphasis
on 'proportional' justice is achieved at the cost of 'creative' justice,
in terms of an individualised service that takes account of special
financial need and of other social needs which can or should be met
by the social services.

Social Security and Welfare

A great many of those who receive benefit need only money and have
no need of any other kind of social service. Among these are a very
large number of the elderly, who receive their allowance as a supplement to their pension. Many such claimants present no problems to
those who administer the scheme and have no need of the attentions
of a social worker. Yet is seems likely that the separation of cash
services from other forms of social service does reduce the likelihood
of attention being given to other aspects of need when the financial
service is offered. The National Assistance Act laid upon the Board
the duty to 'exercise the functions conferred on them by this Act
in such manner as shall best promote the welfare of persons affected

by the exercise thereof'. The Social Security Act of 1966[1] took over this obligation and at the Committee stage of the Social Security Bill the opposition pressed for a more comprehensive welfare responsibility. Miss Mervyn Pike suggested wider powers than those proposed in the Act: the SBC should have 'a duty to seek out those who are, or likely to be, in need of help whether by means of cash or health and welfare services'.[2] (One notes in passing that virtually the whole of this debate was focused on the elderly and it seemed to be assumed that the concept of welfare was irrelevant to any other groups to receive supplementary benefit.) In rejecting the proposed amendment, the then Minister of Pensions and National Insurance, Miss M. Herbison, replied that such a service: 'would require an enormous corps of visiting staff. A wide range of professional skills would be necessary... We must be realistic ... The Committee knows that people of that calibre are not available at present ... Furthermore, much of the work would overlap that of local authorites.' She added, however: '*Welfare does not mean just financial assistance* (my italics) ... We have provided power in the statute to carry on a detection service for both financial and welfare needs.'

Thus responsibility for 'welfare needs' as distinct from purely financial needs was reaffirmed at the point at which the National Assistance Board was taken into a Ministry hitherto solely concerned with the administration of financial benefit. By this time, although still very patchy, local authority personal social services were far more highly developed than had been the case in 1947 and one would have thought the case for such provision less urgent. Interestingly, however—perhaps because society had become so much more aware in the intervening twenty years of the potentialities of social work service—the 1966 debates in the House showed more interest in the 'welfare role' of the then National Assistance Board than had been the case in 1947.

Since 1966 the SBC has sought to define its responsibility in relation to welfare. Despite ministerial pronouncements and the convictions of some officials at higher levels, there is little doubt that the rank and file of officials saw the merger with the Ministry of Pensions and National Insurance and the reduction of certain areas of discretion hitherto vested in visiting officers as an indication of a diminution of interest in 'welfare'—however that was defined. Thus the appoint-

[1] Ministry of Social Security Act, 1966, Para. 3(i).
[2] For these and subsequent extracts, see the second Reading of the Ministry of Social Security Bill, May 1966.

ment of a Social Work Adviser in 1968 was of considerable importance in affirming the importance attached to the welfare function and was viewed with considerable surprise, and some scepticism, at lower levels in the organisation. Much of the writer's work was concerned with the attempt to define this function in relation to the primary task of the SBC in the light of developments in the social services as a whole. More recently, revised and clarified instructions, together with certain developments in training, may have helped to persuade officials at the local level that the phrase in the Act is not an empty one. Its implications are in fact quite complex and far-reaching. At its vaguest, the phrase would seem to suggest that Supplementary Benefit policies must infer respect for the individual. However vaguely expressed, such a responsibility is of profound importance for the system generally and carries with it the obligation to consider the selection of staff and their training in relation to this particular goal as well as to many other aspects of administrative procedures. More precisely, such a phrase raises questions about the detection and referral of needs other than the purely financial, about the way in which claimants who present particular difficulties to the administration are handled, and about the exercise of discretionary financial powers.

The SBC and Welfare Detection and Referral

It is clear that even the 'detection and referral' of other needs places a considerable burden on the SBC. It implies the need for structured liason between the SBC and the relevant social service agencies. It implies that officials should have a sufficient knowledge of people, their needs, and the available services to meet such needs, a sufficient interest to unearth them, and sufficient time to refer and possibly to re-refer. Much, of course, depends on the level of interpretation of the word 'welfare'. At its simplest, it may mean little more, though this is by no means unimportant, than ensuring take-up of welfare foods. A further example of 'practical welfare' might be the referral of the elderly for home help services. The attention of officials is drawn in instructions to many problems for which referral might be appropriate, ranging from bad housing conditions to neglected children or self-neglect in the elderly. Put together, they constitute quite a formidable task for the official, even if such referral is limited to relatively clear-cut matters. Clearly, however, such a function could be much refined and extended to include referral for a whole range of marital and family difficulties. This would raise major difficulties in terms of the skills, training and work loads of the officers. An attempt was made in 1968 to define the responsibility more clearly by relating it to those problems that arose naturally in the course of a thorough financial investigation. That is to say, the commitment to detect and refer was not to be open-ended, although in fact the scope even within the terms of that definition is still wide open to some doubt in interpretation and likely to vary between officials. In addition to limiting the scope, it also implied the need for restraint as a part of respect for the privacy of the individuals concerned. Staff were reminded of the importance of the claimant's wish to be referred, except in certain exceptional circumstances when the welfare of the individual concerned or of children appeared to be at risk. How well or badly this service of welfare detection and referral is in fact carried out is not the point of this discussion. (This issue will be further considered later.) The point to stress here is that the official is expected to take aspects of need, other than the purely financial, into consideration and to take the appropriate steps, even in the many cases which present no difficulties to the Supplementary Benefits administration.

However, it is clear that most difficulties in the separation of financial from other social services arise, not in relation to those for whom some relatively straightforward referral is required, but rather in relation to those whom the writer has elsewhere described, somewhat crudely, as 'the grit in the machine'.[1] These are claimants who, by reason of social or psychological difficulties, present difficulties in the administration of the scheme. They fall broadly into three categories: those who, it is believed by the administration, could work and will not; those who attempt to cheat or abuse the system in other ways; and those who cannot manage on their money. With such claimants the SBC is trapped between its responsibility to protect the public purse and to 'have regard for welfare'. It must seek to persuade men to work; yet there will be some who cannot. It must investigate entitlement (which is not 'a right' until established) and prevent dishonest claims; yet some of those who abuse the scheme are in grave financial or social difficulty. It must have regard to fairness in the granting of discretionary 'extras'; yet there are some whose need is greater because of their inability to manage. With such cases, it is simply unrealistic to talk in terms of a purely financial service which does not take into account related social and psychological difficulties. The development within the SBC of various forms of specialisation,

[1] O. Stevenson, 'The Problem of Individual Need and Fair Shares for All', *Social Work Today*.

C

such as Special Welfare Officers and Unemployment Review Officers, to be discussed later, is part of the strategy devised to cope with these problems. A system of welfare referral breaks down here, not only because of the inadequacy of existing social work services, *but because in some cases no truly just decision concerning benefit can be made without taking into account other elements in the problem.* Thus, in this aspect of the Supplementary Benefits administration, the notion of 'the whole man' may seem more like common sense than a 'blasphemous abstraction'. But it immediately raises the central problem of 'social control' whether by officials or by social workers.

Social Control

Concern about the element of social control in social work appears to be widespread among British social workers at the present time (or is it perhaps an articulate minority?). As has been pointed out, there are many ways in which social workers may exercise social control,[1] ranging from frank, explicit sanctions like rent guarantees to much subtler forms of control, exercised through personal relationship, such as the expression of approval for certain 'desirable' behaviour, for example. In this book it must be examined in relation to the power, actual and perceived, of those who grant money. There can be little doubt that this is potentially one of the strongest elements in enforcing conformity to certain socially approved behaviour. Social workers here and in the States are in the throes of a sharp reaction against the unquestioning acceptance of such a role, exemplified in the bald statement made in 1946 by Meriam:[2]

'To us, it seems undeniable that in a substantial number of cases, families and individuals require more than money . . . They may need guidance from persons possessed of more knowledge than they have; pressure from outside to help them overcome their own inertia; inspiration from persons with visions of possibilities to awake determined ambition. . . .'

He refers to work with individuals:

'not one short inspirational task but prolonged intelligent effort *such as a parent would make with his children*' (my italics).

[1] See O. Stevenson, *New Thinking about Welfare,* Association of Social Workers, 1970.
J. Handler, 'The Coercive Children's Officer', *New Society,* October 1968.
B. Heraud, *Sociology and Social Work,* Pergamon Press, London, 1970.
[2] L. Meriam, *Relief and Social Security,* The Brookings Institution, Washington, 1946.

At such paternalistic sentiments, a shudder runs down the corporate spine of modern social workers. Mayer and Timms,[1] in their recently published account of a group of clients attending a voluntary organisation, have pointed out that, among those who came to the agency for money, few expressed themselves as satisfied with the agency if they did not receive the money they wanted, whatever else in terms of understanding and support they were offered. They also drew attention to the fact that some clients, rightly or wrongly, felt that the granting of money depended on their willingness to discuss their personal problems. Such observations have implications now for British social workers within the existing statutory settings, whose power to give forms of financial and practical help have increased in the last decade, and for the policies, present and future, of the SBC.

The dilemma of the Supplementary Benefits scheme is identified by Titmuss:[2]

'To impersonalise social security programmes, that is, to provide cash benefits as of right with the minimum of forms, rules and regulations can mean a loss of personal contact with consumers . . . Thus opportunities may be lost of 'reaching the hard to reach'; of providing knowledge about other services; of diagnosing unmet needs; of maximising the effectiveness of social policy as a whole. On the other hand, we have to recognise the fundamental importance of providing impersonally and as of right, adequate social security benefits. To the consumer this is an essential freedom.'

Thus Titmuss, whilst presenting the choice, by implication opts for the 'essential freedom' and in so doing will evoke a positive response from different groups: those who remember the indignities of the old Public Assistance in Britain; those who have seen some of the worst aspects of the American system; and those who believe that 'proportional justice' is the safest kind. And yet, one must ask, can this 'essential freedom' be an absolute right if, associated with it, are certain forms of behaviour which, rightly or wrongly, society deems to be undesirable? Freedom is necessarily limited for us all as the price of our interdependence. However, the unequal balance of power that exists between 'the poor' and established authority and the vulnerability of those who depend for their very existence on State resources suggest the need for the utmost caution in any form of 'benefit with

[1] J. Mayer and N. Timms, *The Client Speaks*, Routledge & Kegan Paul, London, 1970.
[2] R. Titmuss, *Commitment to Welfare*, Pantheon Books Inc., New York, 1968.

strings' and for awareness on the part of those who administer it that the recipient is usually the weaker partner in the relationship. (Even this is subtler than at first appears, for a complex relationship exists between the claimant and the official in which on occasions either side may feel powerless—a fact that needs to be understood in relation to the resentment that may build up between them.) This being said, it is nonetheless obvious that the balance of power lies, if not always with the grass roots official, at least within the organisation that administers benefit. Thus the fundamental problem presents itself. On the one hand, it is abundantly clear, as this book will demonstrate, that the problems of some individuals are so intertwined as to make a total separation of financial from other social services not only impracticable but undesirable if their welfare is to be genuinely safeguarded. On the other hand, the control of various aspects of an individual's life via the provision of money must be subject to stringent limitations and careful scrutiny. This does not necessarily mean, however, that it is always improper but that there must be certain safeguards, of which the two most important are: first, that entitlement to *basic* allowances cannot rest, or be believed to rest by claimants, on compliance with what is considered socially desirable behaviour (such as sending the children to school). If there is any 'bargaining' of this kind, it should be in relation to extras. Secondly, the nature of these 'bargains' should be much more clearly understood both by workers (in this case, officials or social workers) and by the clients themselves, so that the implications of the control being exercised are more honestly examined. Such views may at present be unpopular, due to a phase of reaction against the benevolent maternalism of earlier days. In the view of the writer, however, there is no baulking acknowledging the existence of the element of social control in social services and it is through awareness of it, rather than in denial or rejection of it, that clients will be protected from exploitation while considered as individuals with unique and interrelated needs.

In summary, this section has introduced some of the difficulties in theory and in practice of functional unity (as in the usa) and functional separation (as in the uk) of social services administering means-tested benefits and those providing other forms of help. It has been pointed out that within the British system separation is not in fact complete and that, to the extent that it has been achieved, problems of relationship between the separated parts have arisen. The power of those, whether officials or social workers, who administer benefit has been considered as have the dangers inherent in such power. It has, however, been argued that neither official nor social worker can abdicate from 'social control', and that the protection of clients and claimants from its excesses must lie in greater awareness of it. However tendencious the notion of 'the whole man' may at first seem to be, we ignore it at our peril, for it is essential to the administration of creative' justice.

CHAPTER 2

THE EXERCISE OF DISCRETION

Discretion in Public Administration

Reference has been made earlier to the tension that exists between creative (or individualised) justice and proportional (or equitable) justice in the administration of means-tested benefits. Consideration of administrative discretion goes far beyond the Supplementary Benefits Commission and is an important issue in public administration generally—the Comptroller General has commented:[1]

'Fairness ... more often than not is the downfall of the simple rule. Give way to fair play and back they come, those provisos and special conditions, to complicate the rule and spoil the performance. This is particularly so where the government's dealings with the public consists of taking money from those who are thought to have it and paying money to those who are thought to need it.'

'The other reformer is the opposite to the rule simplifier. He wants to remove the rule and substitute discretion. Delegation, we are told, is the thing: give discretion to the man on the spot or to the local office. But ... more often than not the citizen who asks for local discretion only means "give the man on the spot discretion to reach a quick decision so long as he says yes to what I want" '.

Powers of discretion appear to conflict with the traditional view of bureaucracy, propounded by Weber[2] and subsequently refined by Merton.[3] Effective bureaucracy, it was argued, required reliability and strict devotion to regulations. The main characteristics of the system were impersonality and 'routinization' which ensured the efficiency of the operation. However, as Merton pointed out, this had its dangers. Rules might be transformed into absolutes and the subsequent rigidity

---

[1] E. Compton, 'The Administrative Performance of Government', *Public Administration,*

[2] M. Weber, *The Theory of Social and Economic Organisation*, Free Press, New York, 1947.

[3] See, for example, 'Bureaucratic Structure and Personality' in R. K. Merton, *Social Theory and Social Structure*, Free Press, New York, 1968.

could make adaptation impossible when special conditions were encountered. Thus the very element, which in its origins contribute to efficiency, may in certain instances lead to inefficiency. It is to counter just such tendencies that discretion is introduced. These processes have received comparatively little scrutiny until recently although Robson,[1] writing of some of the elements involved in a consideration of justice and administrative law, throws some light on the question. In an admirable analysis he demonstrates the importance of the concept of 'discretion' together with its limitations. He distinguishes between 'consistency' and 'uniformity' and points out that they may on occasions be opposed. 'The idea of uniformity involves the notion of treating alike things which appear superficially to bear a resemblance to one another, regardless of whether they are in fact similar.'

'Consistency presents a *reasoned relation* (my italics) in the first place between decision for the same class of case at different points in time; in the second place between different classes of case at the same point in time; and in the third place between different classes of case at different points in time.

One of the great problems in a modern state is ... how to secure consistency in the field of public administration without creating a mass of rules which actually result in a mere wooden uniformity.

The idea of a discretion which is to be exercised, not in a capricious or impetuous way but in a disciplined and responsible manner, is a conception which has had a wide application in English law and politics. It represents a compromise between the idea that people who possess power should be treated with a free hand ... and the competing notion that contingent control must be retained over them.'

These issues have been further discussed by Hill in a recent book[2]. He points out the importance of distinguishing between maladministration when 'an official uses his discretion to ignore a specific rule' and situations 'in which officials are explicitly required to exercise

---

[1] W. A. Robson, *Justice and Administrative Law*, Stevens, London, 1951.

[2] M. Hill, *The Sociology of Public Administration*, Weidenfeld & Nicholson, London, 1972. For an admirable analysis of some of these issues in relation to the National Assistance Board, see also M. Hill, 'The Exercise of Discretion in the National Assistance Board', *Public Administration*, Spring 1969.

their own judgement ... Confusion arises because the irrefutable or biased use of discretion ... is often mistaken for maladministration.' In general, Hill argues:

> 'It is not the case that discretionary behaviour can easily be eliminated by rules and, moreover, it may in some cases be undesirable ... Some forms of discretion are inevitable in administration; they will be found as a consequence of the complexity of social life, and ethical conflicts endemic within society and the inability of political processes to handle all such conflicts.'

Administrative discretion therefore exists in a state of permanent and not unhealthy tension with its opposite, precisely prescribed rules. Discretionary decisions are those which are based on a judgement of a particular situation, not upon predetermined rules. This does not mean, however, that no official guidance is given as to what factors are to be taken into account in making the judgement which leads to the '*discretionary action*'. That is to say, officials may be given few or many instructions laying down the criteria relevent to the decision. But in the end it is they who must decide in individual cases.

Discretion in the Supplementary Benefits Scheme

What then does discretion involve in the Supplementary Benefits scheme? Discretion may be exercised positively or negatively: that is to say, it may result in the claimant receiving more or less money. Both must be considered in the context of the notion of 'entitlement' to benefit, the basic allowances below which no one may fall. Positive discretion permits flexibility, allows for the possibility of essential requirements that are not met by the fixed scale rates. This may be seen as contributing to individualised justice. On the other hand, it may be argued that there is a sense in which discretionary provisions are aimed at securing proportionalised justice by restoring the claimant to the supplementary benefit level which he would otherwise fall below. It is assumed that, as far as possible, claiments with similar special needs will be treated alike. Negative discretion is in the main concerned with the control of abuse and is essentially the power to delay, refuse or withdraw payment or to give less than usual to prevent exploitation of this scheme. 'Entitlement' must, within a means-tested scheme, be established. Thus doubts exist, in particular in the initial stages of a claim before the facts are verified. Officials are empowered to exercise some discretion as to the amount they pay.

Positive Discretion

The following are some examples of discretionary areas in the Supplementary Benefits administration in which the decision it taken at relatively low levels in the organisation—that is, either by an Executive Officer or his immediate superior. Positive discretion is most commonly exercised in the fields of 'exceptional circumstances additions' (i.e. weekly additions to benefit) and 'exceptional needs payments' (i.e. lump sums). In both fields the SBC's discretion is theoretically unlimited as to amount and unrestricted as to the type of need to be met. In practice the great majority of both weekly additions and lump sums fall into a fairly small number of categories. The most common of the weekly additions are for special diet, extra heating and domestic help; over half the lump sums are for clothing. The SBC have laid down fixed levels for diet and heating, and local officers have standard lists of articles and price lists to guide them in dealing with requests for clothing. Quite large numbers of weekly additions and lump sums are, however, allowed for other needs, such as household equipment and debts, and payments are occasionally made for very unusual purposes, for example, an electric shaver for a half-blind claimant who could not use an ordinary razor without danger.

Prior to the 1966 Ministry of Social Security Act, the numbers of weekly additions were far greater and covered many minor special needs in a very uneven fashion. Discontent about this aspect of the administration led to the introduction in 1966 of a 'long-term addition' to the weekly benefit designed to help those who were receiving a supplementary pension or who had received benefit continuously for two years.[1] Its object was to replace the majority of the weekly additions with regular addition in long-term cases and to cut down the need for minute inquiries into individual special needs. It would not be unreasonable to suggest that the LTA (as it is called) is, in effect, an extra grant for fuel, since this was one of the most frequent expenses for which special additions had been granted and it is likely that the elderly (who are the majority of recipients of the LTA) spend their extra income in this way.

In 1968, when the writer became Social Work Adviser, the impact of these changes was still being felt. This highlighted two important aspects of the exercise of discretion. First, it must be noted that, insignificant as the reduction in discretionary power may seem (especially in comparision with areas to be discussed later), it was a

[1] See Supplementary Benefits Handbook, Para. 51–55.

source of considerable concern and disappointment to officials long established in the National Assistance Board, who saw it (rightly) as a diminution of their responsibility to make choices and thus believed it would reduce the interest and satisfaction of the work. This, as we shall see later, is a factor not to be discounted in successful administration. Secondly, hard on the heels of the legislation, it became clear that the new provisions would not abolish the need for weekly additions; there were still many cases where special needs exceeded the level of the 'long-term addition'. In the first place there were and are those whose special needs continue to be exceptionally high (weekly additions of £1·50 and over are not uncommon). Also, the variety of human needs and of appropriate provision changes over time, both in actuality and in the readiness of services to respond to it. New problems arise demanding new solutions; and yesterday's luxury is today's necessity. The wider application of haemodialysis to patients with kidney disease, for example, has necessitated a very high rate of dietary addition for the cases concerned; and the standards of weekly additions for heating have had to be raised. It seems impossible to conceive of a situation in which positive discretion could be eliminated if a concern for the immense variety of individual needs is to be retained within a means-tested benefit scheme. Titmuss[1] argues strongly for its retention and, in a paper attacking the substitution of the 'rule of law' for administrative discretion, points to the absurdity in which public assistance in New York has found itself by its itemisation of eligibility, following pressure from the 'welfare rights' campaign.

'The increasing application of "legalism" to the public assistance system combined with rising demands for "welfare rights" has led, all over the United States, to a massive fragmentation of entitlement. Itemised legal entitlements, in the assessment of needs and resources, now embrace hundreds of visible articles and objects—practically everything that bedrooms, living rooms, kitchens and lavatories may contain, most normal articles of clothing, day, night, summer and winter, for individuals of both sexes, all ages and nearly all shapes and sizes. For example: in New York City in 1968 (with one million people on public assistance) a man had a "right" to possess one pair of winter trousers at $7.50 (regular sizes); the household has a right to possess in the kitchen one can-opener at 35 cents and, in the

[1] R. Titmuss, 'Welfare, Rights, Law and Discretion', *The Political Quarterly*, Vol. 42. No. 2, April 1971.

lavatory, one toilet tissue holder at 75 cents "but only if your landlord does not have to give you one". And so on and so on through hundreds of itemised entitlements from scrub brushes to panties.

A definition of entitlement in precise material and itemised terms would deprive the recipient of choice, and by prohibiting flexibility would mean that whatever the level of provision it would become a maximum which no official or tribunal could exceed. A legalised itemised prescription of minimum entitlement would become a rigid ceiling against which cases crying out by any human standards for extra help—demanding individualised justice—would press in vain. Nor would such a system eliminate arbitrary decisions—"Your dustbin does not need renewing and your tooth brush is not worn out yet".'

The examples given so far of positive discretion are concerned with exceptional needs and, to a lesser extent, with weekly grants given over and above basic entitlement for exceptional circumstances. This by no means exhausts the possibilities, however, and there are a number of further opportunities for positive discretion in particular situations: for example, whether to award full adult non-householder scale rates to a certain juvenile, such as an unmarried mother. In such a case, the family and financial circumstances of the girl would be relevant in exercising the discretion. Such a distinction might make a difference of up to one pound a week.

Negative Discretion

Negative discretion is also fairly extensive at local office level and is most often applied to unemployed men[1] and separated wives. Most such decisions are concerned with office callers and are intended as temporary measures pending confirmation or clarification of a claimants' statement. It usually involves restriction rather than refusal of payment, for example when a woman declares she had been deserted by her husband but there is reason to doubt the statement. Of course, these powers are potentially dangerous and may in some instances be as liable to abuse as the practices they aim to control Their very existence tends to arouse suspicion in the minds of officers or to suggest to them that higher authority wants them to be suspicious. Therefore the application of negative discretion may be too frequent or may be inappropriately applied as a way of 'playing safe'.

[1] See Chapters 4 and 5.

However, the alternatives must be carefully considered. In the absence of formal sanctions of this kind, it is probable that informal sanctions will increase, such as delaying or discouraging tactics in the payments of allowances. Blau and others[1] have shown how powerful the informal process in bureaucratic systems can be, and it is open to argument that the existence of such formal controls is in fact less dangerous, particularly in matters in which the feelings of officials are aroused.

The Four Week Rule

An example of discretion which has aroused considerable controversy concerns the rule known as 'four weeks and off', whereby a young unemployed single man in an area of high employment may be given a running order for a maximum of four weeks and told that he should be able to find work within that time, will be expected to do so, and that the Commission might refuse further benefit after that period. The *decision* to terminate the allowance is not taken until a man comes back at the end of the four weeks and renews his claim but fails to satisfy an Executive Officer that there is good reason why he has not found work. The geographical areas to which the rule is applied are prescribed by headquarters according to fluctuations in the employment situation. In this there is no discretion at local level. But the local office has instructions not to apply the rule indiscriminately or without regard to the welfare of individuals. Thus there is discretion to exempt certain young men from the rule if its application would result in hardship— for example when mental or physical illness is suspected.[2] In this, as in so many areas of discretion, much depends on the powers of observation as well as on the sympathy of the official concerned, which raises important issues to be considered later concerning selection, training and deployment of officials.

The Cohabitation Rule

Probably the most important single area of discretion which until recently was vested in the visiting executive officer concerns the question of cohabitation. The difficulty and importance of this issue is evidenced by the Commission's decision to publish its second paper

---

[1] P. Blau, *The Dynamics of Bureaucracy*, Chicago University Press, 1955. M. Hill, 'The Exercise of Discretion in the National Assistance Board', *Public Administration*, Spring 1969. P. Blau, 'Orientation Towards Clients in a Public Welfare Agency', *Administrative Sciences Quarterly*, Vol. 5, 1960. J. Jacobs, 'Symbolic Bureaucracy', *Social Forces*, 1969.
[2] See Chapters 4 and 5.

on the subject[1] and will be considered in detail in Chapter 6. Any discussion about discretion as such, however, must be illustrated by reference to the cohabitation rule and the power of the local office to withdraw the order book of a woman believed to be cohabiting. This arises from the statutory regulations which preclude the Commission from paying an allowance to a woman who is living with a man in full-time employment. The presumption is that a man in such circumstances should support the woman and children and that such couples should not be better off, through benefits, than a married couple in similar circumstances. The definition of cohabitation gives rise to much difficulty (although officials are given considerable guidance). Furthermore, if cohabitation is denied and if the 'public acknowledgement' of the situation is not available to guide the official in reaching a decision, a judgement may have to be made that results in the withdrawal of an order book or its voluntary surrender at the time of a visit. It will be appreciated that the line between 'withdrawal' and 'voluntary surrender' is a blurred one, since much depends on the interaction between claimant and official. Thus, discretionary decisions follow a complex process of observation and judgement by the official: for example, the official decides whether to raise the question of cohabitation; he must decide when to press it in the face of denials, and how to interpret an offer to return the orderbook—as an admission of the fact to be accepted or as an angry gesture of defiance to be ignored.

Although the discretionary powers involved in the application of this particular rule are contentious, it seems that, in general, some such powers, within a scheme of means-tested entitlement, are inevitable. It would be ingenuous to suppose that there would not be an increase in the numbers of fraudulent claims if they did not exist. Thus far, therefore, the argument has been in support of the retention of an element of discretion, both positive and negative, within the Supplementary Benefits scheme partly from a concern for individualised justice, partly from the inevitable restrictions on entitlement. This point of view is not, however, currently in favour with more radical social workers.

The Principle of Discretion

Those with knowledge of American public assistance schemes are distrustful of discretionary systems in general and their administration by social workers in particular. Handler, for example, (whose article

[1] *Cohabitation*, HMSO, 1971.

'the Coercive Children's Officer'[1] made a considerable impact in this country) has written interestingly of the ways in which discretionary powers are exercised by social workers in certain public assistance agencies in the USA.[2] On the whole he attacks illiberality rather than inequity. He argues strongly, however, for the separation of social service agencies from public assistance, a point of view which, it will be contended, cannot be taken to extreme lengths without creating a new set of difficulties and injustices. In a sense it is surprising when the criticism of the *principle of discretion* (*as distinct from its operation in practice*), comes from social workers whose general commitment to an ideal of individualised justice has been, one would up to recently have presumed, at the root of their philosophy. It must, however, be acknowledged that the need for discretion arises not only from a concern for unique individual needs but also from the plain fact that resources are never unlimited. As Hill[3] puts it: 'Discretion becomes inevitable at the point where a demand for rationing interlocks with an inability to specify rules upon which such a process can be based.' It is, of course, part of the political process that there should be continuous debate as to whether this point has been reached, whether in fact the resources are properly limited or improperly deployed; whether, for example, the basic allowances of the Supplementary Benefits Scheme are so low as to make exceptional needs grants a necessity for all, rather then an extra for some in particular circumstances. Means-tested schemes are thus particularly likely to contain such elements of discretion since they are by definition a form of 'rationing'. It is beyond the scope of this book to discuss the total allocation of resources to the social services and their division within this sector. But it is only possible to postulate the elimination of discretion from social security if all means-tested benefits were to be abolished. However, in relation to the SBC the constraints are implicit rather then explicit since, as Hill points out, 'SBC officers are not very conscious of actual budgetary limits'[4]—in contrast, for example, to social workers administering the Children and Young Persons Act, 1963.

---

[1] Handler, op. cit.
[2] See, for example, J. Handler and E. J. Hollingworth '*The Administration of Social Services and the Structure of Dependency*', '*The administration of welfare budgets: the views of AFDC recipients*', '*Reforming Welfare: the constraints of the bureaucracy and the client's stigma, privacy and other attitudes of welfare recipients*', Institute for Research on Poverty, Reprints 50, 48, 57, and 66.
[3] Hill, op. cit.
[4] Ibid.

Limitations on Discretion

Support for the principle of discretion, nonetheless, must be qualified in various extremely important ways. These are discussed by Titmuss[1] and fall, in his analysis, under seven main headings:

1. People should be helped to know their rights.
2. The need to reduce or eliminate unnecessary discretionary power.
3. The need to develop sounder and more sensitive quality controls in the administrative process.
4. The need for a continual process of clarification and classification in administrative rule-making.
5. The need for more and better training, retraining, education and staff development programmes.
6. The need for adequate time and adequate facilities.
7. The need to reduce the scope and coverage of means-tested Supplementary Benefits". . . .

Few could dispute the analysis. Any Commission member or administrator is likely to acknowledge the need for these improvements in practice and can point to efforts that are being made. The real difficulty is to assess the point at which the exercise of administrative discretion has fallen so far below a desirable standard as to bring the whole notion into disrepute. In any case, such a view is a matter of judgement on which there would always be differences of opinion. It appears to the writer unlikely that there would be agreement, whether inside or outside the SBC or among particular groups, such as social workers, that, at the present time, the exercise of discretionary powers by Supplementary Benefits officials had reached a point of inconsistency, meanness or prejudice such as to vitiate the intention of the provisions. Nevertheless this is the aspect of the Supplementary Benefits administration most commonly criticised, not only by those whose main academic satisfactions and achievements appear to come from attacking the established system, but also by practising social workers with detailed knowledge of individual cases. This became apparent from an enquiry made of the (then) professional associations of the Standing Conference of Organisations of Social Workers when the writer was Social Work Adviser.[2] (The opinions received

[1] Titmuss, op. cit.
[2] The social workers' relations with the SBC will be discussed more fully in Chapter 9, but since the question of discretionary powers loomed so large in their responses, it is appropriate to consider them in some detail here. The views quoted represent those of the associates who agreed to participate.

were confirmed by a small local survey carried out by the Commission's inspectorate into relations with social workers.)

Social Workers and Supplementary Benefits Discretion

Part of the difficulty arises from social workers' general ignorance of the Supplementary Benefits scheme and their doubt as to what discretionary powers do exist. Most social workers in the inquiry seemed completely uncertain and often in disagreement between themselves as to the kinds of additional expenditure it was reasonable to ask Supplementary Benefits to allow. Thus there was doubt among some as to whether it was possible or appropriate to ask the SBC for bedding, clothing, hire purchase commitments, gas or electricity bills, cost of repairs to houses, and so on. In short, *some* social workers *somewhere* were doubtful as to whether exceptional needs grants could be made for anything for which they were intended, including the most usual ones of bedding and clothing.

The views of the Associations consulted included the following: 'The discretionary powers of the SBC raise problems for social workers partly due to local variations in implementation, and also because some clients seems unable to obtain exceptional needs payments or other benefits without the firm and continuing intervention of a social worker.' Difficulties were frequently encountered over aspects of the SBC's decisions involving discretion and the cause was said to be apparent inconsistency in administration combined with the social workers' imprecise knowledge of the regulations. The judgement of the SBC staff was felt to be affected because they did not understand people with personality disabilities or other psychiatric symptoms, and it is here that the social workers felt they could help. The extent of responsibility of the individual Executive Officer was not known. Some concern was expressed that the introduction of the 'long-term addition' and the other changes in the regulations had apparently reduced the amount of discretion available to individual officers and they had relaxed the vigilance they formerly displayed in ensuring that claimants' needs were met, if necessary by grants for exceptional needs. This view contrasts interestingly with that which urges the reduction of discretion.

As far as the Supplementary Benefits official is concerned, the central problem in a scheme which preserves discretion is well expressed by Hill:

'Officials may differ in the extent to which they regard the official doctrine that the basic allowance should meet all normal expenditure as a tenable one. Similarly, the people in receipt of supplementary benefits differ, in a way not necessarily related to need, in the extent to which they ask for additional or exceptional payments . . . It is natural that the Victorian notions of the deserving or undeserving poor will still have some relevance for decision-making simply because officers often have no satisfactory way of assessing the strength of an exceptional need and will tend to be thrown back on value judgements related to how sensibly the last grant was used etc.'

Hill is, of course, referring here to the exercise of positive discretion, mainly in the field of exceptional needs grants, but the argument stands for the issue as a whole. The inevitability of value judgements in discretionary decisions raises the fundamental question as to how the system can be improved, through staff selection, training and supervision, to minimise the effects of these individual variations. (This will be considered further in Chapter 8.) Titmuss acknowledged this,[1] but the magnitude of the task is daunting. A heavy burden of responsibility is placed upon the sbc to examine, in greater subtlety and depth than has heretofore been evident, the effect of official attitudes on discretionary practices. A defence of the principle of discretion carries with it a moral obligation to improve discrimination and differentiation in its application.

The Publication of Discretionary Powers

One point of controversy, familiar almost to the point of tedium, concerns the publication of discretionary powers. The Commission has consistently refused to publish the actual instructions to officials governing the exercise of discretionary powers. In passing, one remarks the sinister overtones acquired by the phrase 'A' Code. There are, of course, numerous codes used by Supplementary Benefits officials, as by all civil servants, for different purposes. The word 'code' may carry with it for some suggestions of secrecy but it is in common use in the civil service in its original sense of 'a systematic collection of statutes, body of laws so arranged as to avoid inconsistency or overlapping' (Oxford Dictionary). Refusal to publish has been criticised, notably by members of the Child Poverty Action Group.

---

[1] Titmuss, op. cit.

Their case has been strongly argued by Meacher:[1]

'The case for publishing the Supplementary Benefits Commission 'A' Code is not merely one of open government in a democratic society, not even an issue between paternalism and rights in the welfare state, though it closely involves both of these. The case for publication rests squarely on the Ministry of Social Security Act, 1966, which marked the deliberate transition from the meeting of needs to the establishment of entitlement. Yet obtaining benefits under the Act depends at least as much on the unpublished "A" Code rules as on the Act itself and the accompanying Regulations.

If, then, entitlement is to become reality, the rules giving substance to the rhetoric must be made known. Wider issues are involved. Perhaps the most important is that it would begin to reverse the power imbalance between the weak-because-ignorant claimant and the strong-because-knowledgeable social security officer.

At present the weakness of the rules allows stereotype and prejudice in many controversial areas of policy to go unchecked.'

As the preceding discussion has shown, fundamental political issues do indeed arise from the existence of discretionary powers in social security schemes. Furthermore, the degree of 'openness' in their administration, the knowledge of claimants, and those who help claimants, about such powers is a crucial factor. The Commission's growing awareness of this has been demonstrated by the increase in publications which deal, *inter alia*, with discretionary powers. It is clear, however, that much more remains to be done to improve knowledge and understanding of this aspect of the Supplementary Benefits scheme. Publication of codes, as such, seems to the writer a somewhat trivial point from which to attack this problem: manuals of instructions are by definition unsuitable for general consumption. Veiled hints about the sinister contents of the 'A' Code are unconvincing to those whose work has enabled them to peruse it. Indeed, as Hill[1] suggests, the reluctance of the SBC to publish may stem in part 'from the fact that it is a very ambiguous document which sometimes gives clear instructions but often gives merely guidance to officials and in some cases merely sets out the alternatives which officers should consider'. In the writer's opinion, the 'A' Code issue has been exaggerated out of all proportion and has served to confuse rather than highlight the basic and exceedingly important

[1] Hansard, Vol. 827, No. 27, p. 1260 ff.   [2] Hill, op. cit.

matter as to how discretion is in practice exercised and the extent to which the details of its operation should be made public.

In his analysis of the safeguards essential if discretionary powers are to be properly exercised, Titmuss assumes the preservation of the basic structure whereby these powers are vested in the SBC. Such an assumption in relation to the exercise of positive discretion should not, however, go unexamined. The rest of this chapter, therefore, considers the relationship that exists, or might exist, between the SBC and the social work services in this matter.

Discretionary Powers in Social Work

The difficulties inherent in the separation of benefits from other forms of social service were acknowledged by the 1963 Children and Young Persons Act which gave local authority children's departments powers to give cash, in exceptional circumstances, to families when it might 'diminish the need to receive children into care or keep them in care'.[1] This was carried a stage further in the Social Work (Scotland) Act of 1968 which extended these permissive powers to *all* those in need, though with some provisos. The legislation empowers local authorities to:

'promote social welfare by making available advice, guidance and assistance on such a scale as may be appropriate for that area and in that behalf to make arrangements and to provide or secure the provision of such facilities . . . as they may consider suitable and adequate and such assistance may be given to, or in respect of, the persons specified in the next subsection in kind or in cash, subject to subsections 3 and 4 of this section'.

However, the following sections make the provisions more specific. A child under 18 is eligible: 'where such assistance appears to the local authority likely to diminish the need for reception into, or retention in, care'. Any other person is *eligible*: 'where (it) would avoid the local authority being caused greater expense in the giving of assistance in another form *or* where probable aggravation of the persons need would cause greater expense to the local authority on a later occasion'. In either case: 'Before giving assistance to . . . a person in cash . . . a local authority shall have regard to his eligibility for receiving assistance from any other statutory body and, if he is so eligible, to the availability to him of that assistance in his time of need.'[2]

[1] Children and Young Persons Act, 1963. Part II, (ii).
[2] Social Work (Scotland) Act, 1968. Part II, 12 ff.

The Social Services Act of 1970 for England and Wales did not extend the provisions beyond those already granted to the Children's Departments in 1963—a fact worthy of note in view of the Scottish legislation only two years earlier. Since the Supplementary Benefits scheme covers the whole of the United Kingdom, these differences in the powers of social services departments add a further complication to the relations between the two.

The passing of the Chronically Sick and Disabled Persons Act in 1970 strengthens the evidence of a trend to take back into local authority aspects of financial welfare which have hitherto been the responsibility, in the main, of the SBC. Although the Act does not empower any form of direct cash assistance, there are a number of duties placed upon local authorities which would in the past have been regarded as potentially within the scope of the exceptional needs grants of the Commission. For example, local authorities must consider the provision of telephones and of the 'adaptation of the home and additional facilities to secure his greater safety, comfort or convenience'.[1]

All these provisions, imprecisely worded as they are, are of considerable significance. Their existence undoubtedly complicates the relationship between the SBC and local authority social work services. In anticipation of the passing of the Scottish Act, attempts were made by both parties to define respective responsibilities. However, it would seem that in practice these attempts have not been altogether successful and more recent clarifications of policy behaviour the SBC and the new Social Service departments in local authorities in England and Wales may fare no better, despite excellent intentions.[2] This is not to imply that the clarifications are useless. The plain fact is, however, that the vagueness of the powers on both sides means that, in the last resort, many decisions must be taken at local levels on a judgement of an individual situation, and that local relationships will affect such judgements. Thus, for example, the occasions on which the SBC rather than a Social Service Department will clear a rent or fuel debt to prevent eviction, continue to be at times a source of dispute.

Casework and Financial Discretion

A situation in which responsibility for casework and responsibility

[1] Chronically Sick and Disabled Persons Act, 1970. Para. 2, (i).
[2] Unpublished memoranda on this subject were circulated widely to the relevant persons.

for certain discretionary financial powers are totally separate, will never be satisfactory. The social worker is free to press for financial help for a particular individual or family without regard to the wider implications of such a provision, in particular to the effect on others in the locality. The lack of accountability to the agency means that there cannot be the same sense of involvement in recommending a grant. The official, disassociated from the planning for the general welfare of the individual or family, at the receiving end of requests for financial aid and accountable to his superiors, is likely to be—or to be seen to be—distrustful of requests from social workers. Thus are stereotypes created: the social worker, the giver, the indiscriminate champion of the poor; the official, the withholder, the guardian of the public purse. It must be emphasised that these *are* stereotypes; but like all such, they contain an element, albeit distorted, of the truth and are undoubtedly part of the mythology which each has of the other, thus contributing to the discomfort in the relationship. Although they may also be seen in relationships between administrators and social workers within the *same* organisation, they are more acute and less resolvable between social workers and the SBC, because of the organisational separation. In many ways, it has suited social workers well since they have had a constitutional preference for giving rather than refusing, for acting the benign rather than the rejecting parent. The structure enables British social workers to evade the less congenial aspects of the service which their colleagues in (for example) Israel and the USA still carry. Yet the separation of services affects the welfare of claimants. That this is so was borne out in the enquiries made during the writer's period as Social Work Adviser. There are a number of reasons. First, and perhaps most striking, social workers were often reluctant to approach the SBC on behalf of clients for discretionary grants. It is impossible to know whether this was justified apprehension in the face of previous refusals or whether a 'mythology of meanness' had come to surround the SBC. Secondly, when approaches were made, there was often a sense of frustration on both sides. For the official, there was, on occasion, doubt about the validity of the request, sometimes because the total family situation was not as fully understood as by the social worker but sometimes also because facts about family resources were known *more* fully. Sometimes there was an underlying lack of confidence in the social worker's objectivity. For the social worker, there was resentment at having to 'make a case' out to officials who were not professionals. Perhaps even more important than this—for after all most social workers have to justify their requests to administrators within their own agencies—was the feeling of making an approach to an alien organisation whose structure and personnel were for the most part, unfamiliar. In short, the problem was not of communication between enemies but between strangers. Small wonder, therefore, if on occasions the clients suffered through the inability of the respective parties to clarify their positions.

Who Should Exercise Discretion?

What is the remedy? Greater responsibility in social work for financial assistance may seem a retrogressive step. Past experience and the experience of other countries indicates that, questions of principle apart,[1] social work develops in depth and in scope when it is freed from the obligation to relieve purely financial need. Yet responsibility for the administration of basic entitlement is not the same as possessing discretionary powers. It would be possible to envisage three different patterns from that which at present is developing, which seems confused and uncertain.

First, positive discretionary powers might be removed from the SBC altogether and given to social workers, leaving the SBC to administer entitled benefits only according to precise rules. Secondly, the relationship between social workers and Supplementary Benefits might be re-defined so that the recommendation of the social worker on such matters might be automatically accepted. Thirdly, the administration of discretion within Supplementary Benefits might be changed so as to include within the system greater expertise in what we have called 'individualised justice'. This might imply greater use of social work skills within the SBC.

All these suggestions, however, carry with them the implication of greater power for the social worker in relation to finance. As has been discussed in the first chapter, this raises many questions about the exercise of social control through such functions. However, even if such developments were accepted as a legitimate extension of social workers' power, it is evident that British social workers have much to learn about this. The recent study by Heywood and Allen[2] of the uses made by four Childrens Departments of their discretionary powers under the 1963 Children and Young Persons Act demonstrates that there is much confusion and uncertainty as well as wide variations between authorities in the use made of such powers. Clearly both the

[1] See Chapter I.
[2] J. Heywood and B. Allen, *Financial Help in Social Work*, Manchester University Press, 1971.

value systems underlying the practice and a greater understanding of the place of discretionary help within the total plan for professional help to particular clients needs to be much more fully explored. At present there is a risk that increased power by social workers in this field will satisfy neither the principles of equitable justice nor those of creative justice; neither the virtues of the good bureaucrat nor that those of the truly professionalised worker will be sufficiently developed. There are many social workers in post at present with less training and less skill than officials in the exercise of discretion.

In any case, many discretionary grants do not involve or need the intervention of a social worker. All this being said, however, the fact remains that the essence of social work skill lies in the capacity to look at a family or individual problem in the round as an interaction of social, psychological and material need; there are a number of cases in which such skills seem to the writer to be essential, if public funds are to be used neither wastefully nor meanly but appropriately, and if the individual is to be helped as fully as possible. This is said in full acknowledgement of the element of social control involved. But it seems better that the aim should be to exercise control openly by those who are presumed to be—and one hopes increasingly will be—trained to consider the problem in a manner impossible and inappropriate for Supplementary Benefits officials. The number of cases is small in relation to Supplementary Benefits work as a whole, especially if one includes the elderly. But among those who need social work help there will be a large number for whom, at some time or another, discretionary grants or allowances will be necessary.

Removal of Positive Discretion from the SBC

So which of the three suggestions might be followed? To remove positive discretionary powers from the SBC would be a radical and extreme step. The granting of certain discretionary powers to local authorities, however, could be seen as the thin end of a wedge. It will be extremely interesting to see whether in fact these powers are increasingly used to avoid the element of confrontation between organisations in the present system. It is certain that if these powers are seen by local authority committees to be used by social workers more and more for purposes which are within the statutory ambit of the SBC, questions will soon be asked and battles will ensue above the heads of the social workers. In any case it is important to consider the implications of such an arrangement for the welfare of clients. If a transfer of all discretionary powers were made, a heavy extra burden of work would be placed upon social workers in relation to clients, many of whom did not need the services of a social work department for any other reason. It would involve the claimants in a separate approach to social workers which might be complicated, would on occasions be resented and might deter claimants from applying. Local authorities might vary in their practice more than the SBC. Lastly, and very important, it would take away the element of positive discretion from officials whilst leaving elements of negative discretion involved mainly in the control of abuse. Thus the role of Supplementary Benefits officials would not, and could not, become purely bureaucratic but its controlling, even punitive, aspects would be emphasised at the expense of concern for welfare. An advantage would be that applications for discretionary grants would enable a proper investigation of related needs, especially in the case of the disabled or elderly. At present, there is a strong possibility that, despite a system of 'welfare referral', financial needs will be treated in isolation. How else to account for the fact, for example, that so little has been known until recently about the numbers and needs of the disabled, large numbers of whom were in receipt of supplementary benefit? However, it could be argued that this could be overcome by a general improvement within the Supplementary Benefits system. On the whole it would seem that the arguments against such an arrangement are strong, both from a long-term theoretical standpoint and in relation to the practicalities of the current British scene. Nevertheless, the inconsistencies of the present division of responsibilities and their implications for future developments need to be carefully watched. It is quite possible that the SBC will welcome a decrease in these responsibilities with the resultant financial saving without recognising the long-term effects on its service, in particular on attitudes of officials, and on the general pattern of social security and social work.

Social Workers' Recommendations

The second possibility would be to accept the recommendation of the social worker for discretionary allowance in cases in which he is involved. The situation at present is confused. Some discretionary allowances are within the authority of an Executive Officer to grant and it is evident that they vary greatly in the weight they give to the social worker's recommendation. (There is no clarification of this point in their instructions.) This would not involve administrative change and has the merit of organisational simplicity. It would not eliminate positive discretion from the role of the Supplementary

Benefits official since large numbers of claimants requiring such help would not be on the social worker's books. It is probable that the cases in which the social worker's recommendation had to be accepted would be, by and large, those with which the official is likely to have least sympathy—the 'voluntarily unemployed' for example. This, it could be argued, supports the suggestion if it meant that such claimants get a fairer deal. On the other hand, there would clearly be the danger —indeed the virtual certainty—that cases would arise in the same area (the same street, the same block of flats) in which two claimants, one in touch with a social worker, the other not, received different treatment in very similar circumstances. Both agencies might be acting entirely properly within their different terms of reference, but the resulting inequities might well be marked and sometimes conspicuous. Such an arrangement, moreover, would also have the effect of polarising the situation still further. Negative discretion would be retained and there is the possibility that resentment on the part of officials at having to accept such a recommendation would show itself in treatment of the claimants in other contexts—for example, pressure on those considered to be 'voluntarily unemployed', or denying cohabitation. That the majority of officials are fair-minded and reasonably objective cannot blind us to their human failings. To be denied responsibility, to be required to give without understanding is a sure recipe for resentment. One must add to this the dangers for the social worker in the lack of accountability to his own organisation for the recommendation. Accountability and responsibility reinforce each other and it is unlikely that social workers would exercise due restraint in such an arrangement, even when—as is far from being achieved at present— social work is a fully qualified profession. Indeed, given the present separation of function, it is likely that the fully qualified professional is more intolerant of limits, more wholehearted in his championing of the underdog, less interested in protecting the public purse than his colleague who has not been so trained. This raises the question as to whether this tension over discretionary power between social workers and Supplementary Benefits officials is healthy and beneficial, preserving a necessary balance. In the opinion of the writer, the tension is necessary and healthy but one which should be contained within the organisations and individuals, not dichotomised between (in this case) the opposing forces of Supplementary Benefits and local authority social service departments. In any case, automatic acceptance of social workers' recommendations would create a particularly dangerous situation in which one party—the official—was powerless in the here-and-now but powerful at other times, in relation to the same claimant. Thus it would seem that despite its superficial attractiveness, this second possibility is a dangerous one.

Social work within the SBC

The third suggestion of increasing expertise in human relations within the SBC has a number of different aspects, the selection and training of Supplementary Benefits staff, and the degree of specialisation in local offices being two of the most important. Suffice it to say here that it is, in the opinion of the writer, essential to devise some form of local office specialisation in which certain officials, suitably selected, trained and deployed, are given designated responsibility to cooperate with social workers on matters involving the exercise of discretion—*positive and negative*—in relation to the social worker's clients. If this exists at present, it is by the exercise of local initiative and is informal although local offices have been encouraged to make such arrangements. Moreover, it may conflict with other demands of the organisation. Certainly, it is impossible to conceive of a satisfactory solution to the problem without such an arrangement.

This would not, however, eliminate the need for some social work expertise within the Supplementary Benefits scheme to support local offices in such developments and to establish confidence among social workers that they have a channel for professional communication. This has been acknowledged by the SBC in the appointment of a permanent Social Work Adviser and the decision to appoint Regional Social Work Officers. (There are twelve regions, serving about 420 local offices.) It is clear that such a structure could be of great importance in establishing machinery for effective communication between the SBC and social work and for consideration of cases of particular difficulty. However it is important to clarify the purpose of such appointments which might otherwise be interpreted as implying the intention of the SBC to develop social work alongside, or even in competition with, existing social work services. This is not so. Such appointments simply acknowledge, *inter alia*, that discretionary powers cannot be exercised properly if there is a complete separation of the Supplementary Benefits administration from social work, which leads to polarisation of attitudes and works to the detriment of individuals in need. An increase, however small, in the numbers of social workers within the Supplementary Benefits scheme may help to provide a better balance between proportional and creative justice within the administration. Much depends, however, on whether the social work profession can sort out and define its position on the 'social control' issue and whether it can demonstrate increasing expertise in the use of discretionary grants as part of treatment plans. This is not to deny that there are many situations in which the need is straightforward and purely financial. In such cases, it has been argued, the expertise of the Supplementary Benefits officials, provided it is informed by appropriate attitudes, should suffice. In those cases, however, in which the *problem itself* is compounded of social, psychological and practical elements, the skills of the social worker, as yet uncertain and immature, seem to offer the best chance of justice. Their use *within* the SBC to communicate *within and across* systems seems worth trying.

CHAPTER 3

THE STRUCTURE AND ORGANISATION OF THE SUPPLEMENTARY BENEFITS ADMINISTRATION

This chapter assumes unfamiliarity with the basic structure and organisation of Supplementary Benefits administration. No doubt there will be some readers for whom it is unnecessary. It is clear, however, that for many social workers this is unknown territory and this, combined with the usefulness of the description for overseas readers, justifies time spent in such an outline. For without such knowledge it is impossible to discuss sensibly the problems of relationship between the Supplementary Benefits Commission and social workers. It is the impression of the writer that, in many of the criticisms levelled at the Supplementary Benefits Commission, psychological reasons for the difficulties are imputed when it would be more profitable to examine them in sociological terms. In particular, descriptions of the attitudes of officials as punitive or indifferent may or may not be accurate in certain instances; but if they leave out of account facts about the way the work is organised and the roles the officials are required to assume —which may be of equal or greater relevance—their usefulness is limited. The description that follows does not aim to be comprehensive. Rather it picks out those aspects of organization which are of particular relevance to the theme of this book.

Local Offices

A local Supplementary Benefits office is organisationally more akin to a factory production line than to a social work department. It is geared to the payment of money, as reliably, quickly and efficiently as possible. It is quite a large-scale exercise, involving payments amounting to over £600 million each year. A substantial part of the work behind the scene is concerned with the renewal of order books and, in 'the caller' section, with immediate payment to meet need. Thus the central aim of the organisation, which is in principle much simpler than that of a social work department also gives the clue to a problem in relation to social workers' clients. Unfortunate as it may be, it is nevertheless inevitable that within such an organisation—geared to 'high productivity', keen to streamline procedures and under considerable pressure—the difficult or exceptional case may be to some degree resented. This, implicitly at least, is felt not to be the main business of the organisation and interrupts the flow of work. (On the other hand it may be welcomed as a relief from routine.) The closer links with social insurance payments following the merger with the Ministry of Pensions and National Insurance have increased such tendencies. However these should not be seen solely or predominantly in negative terms for the advantages of the growing concern with management and organisational techniques in such a crucial sector of the public service does not have to be argued. One simply needs the proviso that such techniques must make allowance for the interruptions to the work flow occasioned by claimants who present difficulties—which has an important bearing on the way local offices are organised.

Executive and Clerical Officers

Executive Officers in the local office are regarded as the key men. An Executive Officer (EO) in the civil service is either in charge of a group of Clerical Officers (COS) and Clerical Assistants (CAS) or handles the investigation of claims beyond the scope of the CO. Much of this investigation for supplementary benefits is done by EOs because of the significance attached to it. COS do less important investigations and interviews and some supervision of CAS. CAS do mainly routine work like filing, writing postal drafts and record-keeping, and trace the case-papers of people who have claimed before. The general outdoor duties of the EO (as distinct from specialised duties to be discussed later) are to pay the first home visits following a claim; to make further visits to certain categories of case regarded as more complicated than most, whether routine or exceptional; and to make the necessary calculations and authorisations for payment. Traditionally, each EO has covered a particular geographical area and has been known as a 'Territorial Executive Officer', (TEO). Within that area and within certain administrative limits, he has had a considerable measure of autonomy. Within a particular geographical area a group of Clerical Officers also pay home visits. Their duties consist of visits, routine or exceptional, to categories of case considered to be less complicated. Clerical Officers are not accountable to the TEO. In general, they work under EOs specially designated to supervise their visiting or involved in assessment. There have been and continue to be experiments in varying this arrangement. Once such gave the function of recommendation of payment to a different 'indoor' EO so that TEO simply gathered the facts. The arguments for this were largely organisational, in terms of the efficiency derived from greater job-specialisation. But the loss of autonomy was regretted by the TEOs and the expected rise in efficiency did not occur. Although arguments continue within the SBC as to the merits of the TEO system and experiments in varying the pattern continue, it remains the usual method of deploying 'outdoor' EOs. It should be noted that the structure does not facilitate formal contact between the TEO and the visiting Clerical Officer about individual claimants whom they both know.

The 'indoor' EO of most importance in direct service to the public is responsible for 'the caller section' of the office. He interviews some claimants but the bulk of the interviewing is done by Clerical Officers who must report their findings to him.

In any local office, therefore, the group of EOs and COs and the relations between them is of crucial importance in determining efficiency and attitudes. Formally, the greater authority of the EO is clearly defined. However, as always, informal factors have to be taken into account. Shortages of EOs have meant that a number of COs are 'acting up' as EOs. Turnover of staff may mean that a number of COs are much more experienced than any of the EOs—which is bound to affect their relationships. In any case, the COs who check the factual accuracy of decisions act as an unofficial brake on the power of the EO who knows that his decisions will be scrutinised and discussed. Perhaps most important of all, the EO, if he has not seen the claimant himself, is dependent on the CO, not only for the accuracy of information upon which to base a recommendation, but also in more subtle ways, when discretionary powers are involved. It is obvious that the way a request from a claimant is presented by the CO, for example the amount of supporting evidence that is produced, may have an effect on the EO's decision. This has some rather disquieting implications in the light of information and opinions obtained while the writer was in the SBC for it was clear that the formal allocation of responsibility made the EO more anxious and therefore more motivated to learn so that he might make 'good' decisions, than was the CO. Of course other factors enter into this. It may in part be related to lower educational and intellectual standards although this is by no means clear. It is almost certainly related to the fact that a greater number of COs take the post for convenience—married women wanting to be near home, for example—and have neither career ambition nor a specific interest in this work. While the latter may also be true of the EO whose entry to the SBC rather than, say, to the Ministry of Defence may have been fortuitous, his choice of the civil service as a career will make an interest in career prospects probable. All this being said, however, it seems likely that the COS' official lack of responsibility for decision-taking is an important factor in keeping motivation to learn low, which affects training programmes and will be considered further later. After discussion with many clerical officers one was forced to conclude that, for many, there was little desire to question why.

Senior Local Office Officials

Many local offices have two senior officials—a Higher Executive Officer (usually styled Deputy Manager) and a Senior Executive Officer (the Manager). Some smaller offices have an HEO in charge. Some larger offices, especially those that have integrated with the insurance side of the department, have higher posts for those in charge. These senior officials are vitally important in the detailed day-to-day organisation of a complex system and in setting the tone of the office in regard to staff morale, attitudes to claimants and so on. Of course, the Manager works with many constraints and according to prescribed regulations in many aspects of the organisation. Nevertheless, the degree of delegation does allow for experiment and innovation, which is essential because of the variations in local conditions—for example in the number of callers, categories of claimant on the total load of the office (old people, unemployed, etc.), ease or difficulties in recruiting Clerical Officers and Assistants, staff turnover and so on. There are a multiplicity of ways in which the details of administration need to be varied and in which they affect the smooth running of the office. It is, *par excellence*, a management task, requiring skills very different from those of a civil servant comparable in grade within the SBC, engaged in decision-making related to specific cases, although this too must on occasions fall to the lot of the Manager. In addition to the managerial role, senior officials will, of course, be required to take decisions on certain issues referred upwards by EOs, following the normal conventions of the civil service. Thus, the SBC has recently instructed that decisions to withdraw an order book from a woman believed to be cohabiting must be taken by a senior officer in the local office. One must, however, draw a distinction between those cases in which referral upwards is mandatory—as that just described—and those in which it is left to the discretion of the EO to ask for advice. Mandatory referral upwards can, of course, be avoided by taking a decision that avoids doing something exceptional. As far as the informal referral is concerned, much will depend on the personalities and experience of the officials involved, their mutual trust and the informal machinery of consultation which has been developed. As with relations between EOS and COS, many decisions of direct relevance to the welfare of clients will be affected by relationships and structures of a less formal kind, as well as by the willingness or reluctance of the official to complicate life for himself by making formal submissions.

The Visiting of Claimants

The most usual reasons for the visiting of claimants are: first, to establish entitlement; secondly, to review allowances in the light of changes of circumstance; thirdly, to investigate reported changes in circumstances. Other reasons are: to investigate applications for exceptional needs payment and advice; and to check cases where abuse is suspected. In all visiting, as in office interviews, there is a general obligation to see if there is a need for welfare referral action. But this is not, of course, the primary objective of the visit.

A very large number of visits are those which are described as 'review visits', to investigate possible changes of circumstance in those whose entitlement has been established. It is not always appreciated that, for such, visiting frequencies are laid down in instructions and that the decision as to how and when to visit is not within the discretion of the official to the same degree as for social workers. The instructions lay down the frequency of visiting according to certain categories of case: broadly speaking, the decision as to frequency is taken either on grounds of welfare or on grounds of suspicion of abuse. As instructions stand, the longest time a case can go unvisited as part of regular review routine is two years—to an old person living in a home or with relatives, for example. The shortest time is three months —to one-parent families, for example. However, it is within the discretion of the TEO to visit more frequently, even weekly in special circumstances. There has been much discussion within the SBC about the value of review visiting. It has been argued that it is uneconomic to provide an extensive service to check on changes of circumstances; that few claimants are dishonest and most are capable of providing written statements sent by post that would ensure proper variations in the allowance. Claimants are required to notify changes of circumstance as they occur but when they do not do so, the infrequency of visiting, especially in the case of the elderly, means that, despite official exhortations to notify changes, many are deprived of increases due to them for a considerable period, and not all are paid retro-spectively. Furthermore, even the prescribed frequencies have not been adhered to, such has been the pressure on staff. At one time visiting was tied to order book renewal. When the visit could not be paid at the appropriate time, it was waived altogether so that it was not uncommon for the scheduled time to be doubled. The changes in home-visiting already mentioned should put an end to this state of affairs and prevent claimants being out of contact with local offices perhaps for years at a time. The remedy adopted is to introduce a system of postal communication at yearly intervals for all cases which do not present special problems or potential problems, subject to the safeguard of a visit being made wherever the claimant shows he is unable to fill in the form sent to him. Experiment with the new system suggests that the majority of claimants are able to complete the necessary forms satisfactorily. The advantage of the new system is hoped to be that visiting will in future be reserved for those cases where it is essential to the proper discharge of the Commission's functions, including their welfare function. The new arrangements take account of the development of local authority services since the Commission's welfare function was discussed in the House of Commons Debate on the 1966 Social Security Act, and also take account of the impracti-cability of arranging for large numbers of pensioners to be visited frequently enough for their changing needs to be recognised. However, it remains to be seen whether the reduction of routine visiting will lead, in fact, to more effective visiting of the few.

The purpose of the foregoing discussion has been to give, in brief, a picture of the way in which a local office functions. To those readers who are social workers, it will be immediately apparent that the organisation conforms much more closely to the traditional style of bureaucracy than does a social work department, although the exercise of discretion, discussed fully in Chapter 2, is clearly a more significant element in the work than it is in some civil service departments. However, it is most important for social workers to appreciate that a great proportion of time is spent on factual and routine activity connected with establishing and varying entitlement: this is the primary task. It gives the local office its characteristic style and is one in which the concerns of social workers may seem peripheral.

The Hierarchy

Local offices are, of course, part of a wider structure. There are twelve Regional Offices, including the Scottish and Welsh Central Offices,

E

which in turn relate to the London Headquarters of the Department of Health and Social Security. It is beyond the scope of this book to discuss these relationships in any detail, except to draw attention to the difficult balance that has to be struck between local office or regional autonomy and central control. This issue affects many aspects of the administration from organisational experiment to discretionary decisions on individual cases. It highlights a problem created by the transfer of functions from local authorities to the NAB. In the commendable desire for national consistency, a tension was inevitably created between the need for speedy decision-making at a local level and the risks of inconsistency inherent in such delegation. In fact, the problems go deeper than those of consistency, for the degree of responsibility given to officials at different levels in the organisation affects the morale of the service and in turn the way the public is served. But the dangers are obvious. The officials of the SBC are accustomed, as are all civil servants, to work in a more structured and hierarchical organisation than are social workers. Their relationships are in the main uncomplicated by 'the professional element' which is the source of so much conflict amongst social workers in, for example, a local authority social service department. This fact is of relevance in relationships between the two. By and large the civil servant has been trained not to question (at least openly) the decisions of his superiors. Whatever private reactions there may be, the roles are so structured, especially in the lower grades, that authority is accepted without much challenge. There is, of course, relief as well as resentment in such a position because such organisation puts the onus for particular decisions 'up the line'. In fact it is likely that an official might not resent as much as would a social worker a reversal of his previous decision whether by a superior officer, by an Appeal or a complaint to an MP. This is not to underestimate the strength of feeling that may be engendered in particular situations. It is to point out, however, an important distinction between a professional and a bureaucratic orientation, a distinction which may on occasions be sharpened by the fact that some professionals have a greater emotional investment in their work.

The Evolution of Policy

Insofar as individual cases are concerned, the role of Headquarters is to make decisions where issues of precedent or particular difficulty are involved. Certain problems must, by definition, be referred to Head Office. Thus, for example, a decision to pay the fare of an immigrant back to his native country can only be taken at Headquarters, as can some decisions to prosecute.[1] In other cases, however, upward referral is one of the ways by which variations in individual circumstances are examined to see whether they are unique and demand particular discretionary decisions or whether they raise issues of policy and demand alteration of the existing regulations or instructions. The importance of such machinery is obvious and relevant to the discussion of discretion. For this is the way in which the administration retains its flexibility and gathers information so as to formulate general rules, which are in a constant process of revision and often based upon a redefinition of need.

That this process within the Supplementary Benefits administration is analagous to that within a social work organisation or within any other organisation concerned with the evolution of social policy is obvious. It is stressed here for that very reason—the Supplementary Benefits organisation is an important element in the evolution of social policy. It is the writer's impression that few social workers appreciate the significance of the role of senior civil servants at Headquarters level in this. Innumerable issues directly affecting the welfare of claimants, many of which arise in the first instance from referral of specific cases, receive the most detailed scrutiny. However— and this is relevant to later consideration of the contribution of social work to the Supplementary Benefits administration—senior officials can only make decisions on individual cases on the basis of information passed up the line. They may, of course, ask for more. But knowing what to ask is in itself a skill in relation to those problems to which social and psychological factors are relevant to the decision taken and one which it cannot be assumed officials will possess.

An actual example known to the writer was an application by a psychiatrist for payment of the fare of a married immigrant woman back to her own country. She had frequent and serious spells of mental illness. In such a case, in which the welfare of the claimant is of overriding statutory importance, this was a fact that troubled officials greatly in reaching a decision. Certain questions needed to be asked concerning her immediate family situation, for example, about her marriage and her husband's wishes in the matter; the age of the children, their ties to their parents, and the possible effects on them of the decision. Other questions needed to be asked about the social

---

[1] Such upward referral is not, of course, the *only* way by which Headquarters obtains knowledge for policy development. See, for example, p. 68 for reference to the role of the Supplementary Benefits Inspectorate.

circumstances to which the women might be returning and what it was hoped to gain by the arrangement. To form a judgement and take a decision on such an issue requires not only facts but an understanding of what information is needed and a sifting and interpretation of a complicated family situation. Similarly, complex background information is required in cases in which prosecution for 'refusal to maintain' is contemplated, that is to say, cases in which a man, thought to be capable of work, is refusing it and receiving Supplementary Benefits. Senior officials are aware that cases coming to their notice are a very biased sample, but they play their part in the general study of trends and developments reported by Regions, and in particular by the Commission's Inspectorate,[1] who are an important means of keeping in touch with the administration of the scheme at local level.

The Social Work Adviser

Of significance also to the role of Headquarters is the post of Social Work Adviser. In creating the permanent post, the Commission saw the main tasks as contribution to training and the promotion of liaison with the personal Social Services; and as helping to set up a social work element in the Commission's Regional Offices. The post was established in the Department's Social Work Division, which was shortly afterwards combined with the Home Office Children's Inspectorate to form the new Social Work Service. As Social Work Service Officers are appointed to Supplementary Benefits Regions they, as members of Social Work Service, work under the professional direction of the Social Work Adviser; in their capacity as members of the Commission's Regional Staff they are responsible to the Regional Controller.

The permanent Social Work Adviser works closely with all the policy divisions of Supplementary Benefits Headquarters and is involved, directory or indirectly, with the various common service branches, for example those concerned with staff training, instructions (the 'Codes') and in research. The Adviser's relationships with the Regions will develop further with the appointment of the Social Work Service Officers, currently being appointed by the Dept. of Health and Social Security.

The Supplementary Benefits Commission

To conclude this discussion of the general working of the scheme,

[1] A small group of officials whose task is to investigate and report directly to the Commission on many different aspects of the work.

reference must be made to the Commission as such which, in 1966, replaced the National Assistance Board, set up in 1947. Such a body might be expected to play a part in keeping the administration of the scheme separate from party politics and the 1966 Social Security Act which merged the old NAB with the Ministry of Pensions and National Insurance preserved the principle of an independent statutory body in creating the SBC. The Commission is primarily concerned with questions of entitlement to supplementary benefits, although it is also a statutory authority for other means-related benefits.[1] (The administration of the Family Income Supplement is a further recent responsibility.) It also has responsibilities for Reception and Re-establishment Centres, and for the Polish hostel at Ilford Park.[2] However, in the Supplementary Benefits Scheme itself, the Commission is much involved in its broad direction and with administration as well as adjudication. As such it is concerned with resources and priorities and must be in touch with the whole of the Department's services that bear on the administration of the scheme. This fact, and their own career experience, means that the Commission provides a source of informed and independent advice within the Department. Their collective experience is wide and may include trade union practice and many aspects of the social services. They are independent—they cannot be in the House of Commons—and this also means that, since they do not change with governments, they provide an element of continuity and complement the knowledge of the permanent officials and the independent advice from sources outside the Department.

The status of the Commission is, however, somewhat ambiguous since it sits within the Department of Health and Social Security, served by the civil servants of that Department, and in a somewhat delicate relationship with the Minister of the day. In its advisory role, it is bound at times to negotiate rather than to cooperate with the Minister. It does not fit readily into conventional ideas of ministerial responsibility and may therefore be a source of confusion if not of suspicion as to where power really lies. Despite this, however, the writer's impression is that it performs a useful function in bringing independent and critical minds to bear on issues of great social importance. If these views are not accepted by the Minister, the care with which they have been formulated, and the standing and independence of the persons involved, make it likely that they will receive serious consideration. Such a body could, of course, become a tool of the

[1] See DHSS Report, 1970, Chapter 2, pp. 95, 100–2.
[2] DHSS Report, 1970, Chapter 2, pp. 99–100.

established civil service whose skilled manipulations (albeit well-intentioned) of lay committees are well known and no different from those of social workers in local government. However the permanent embarrassment to Ministers of having an obviously rubber stamp Commission would probably be far greater than the temporary embarrassment of disagreement on a particular issue. Individual appointments are obviously crucial in this as is the trust and understanding created between Commission members and senior officials. The impression gained by the writer in the period in which she was Social Work Adviser was that the Commission's influence was considerable. Certainly the involvement of Commission members was no mere formality and there was general commitment and concern about the objectives and the problems of the scheme.

Commission members meet monthly. Most aspects of the Supplementary Benefits scheme ranging from policy on particular matters, for example, payment of high rents, to matters of organisation such as the substitution of Giro orders for cash payments, are presented to the Commission for discussion and recommendation. The interaction of Ministers, Commission Members and senior civil servants is, however, continuously changing and the real (as distinct from the formal) nature of these relationships must obviously be a matter for continuous concern if the Commission members are to affect the evolution of social policy in such an important area as supplementary benefits.

Specialisation

We move now to consider the question of specialisation within the Supplementary Benefits administration at local office and regional levels.[1] The specialisations that will be discussed are essentially 'specialisations by task' rather than those that carry special skills or expertise. They have evolved as a result of concern that certain aspects of the work needed more time and attention than the officer on general duties could give and imply a decision that these aspects of the work could be carried out more efficiently and constructively if attention was focused on them by one specially designated officer. The varieties of specialisation to be considered here are all of equal grade, namely Executive Officer; thus the administration does not grant any superiority to those who accept these particular roles in the organisation, although such a specialist post will normally help in an officer's career. For social work readers, this is an important distinction since specialisation may suggest the kinds of skill and expertise associated,

[1] See Chapter 8 for a discussion of developments in training for specialisation.

for example, with the medical profession. In fact, as will be shown, there is some confusion within the Supplementary Benefits administration on this issue. It is, of course, inevitable that those who specialise in a particular task will acquire a certain facility in it and it may often be necessary to provide a form of training for it. There comes a point, however, when particular tasks require skills that go beyond the conventional 'tricks of the trade' and that may be described as professional or semi-professional. The outstanding example of this within the SBC is the Special Welfare Officer whose tasks will be discussed in greater detail in Chapter 7. The swo is, in the opinion of the writer, required to fill a role indistinguishable from a social worker although he needs, in addition, expertise in the Supplementary Benefits scheme. For many years, however, the job was presented as one that was necessary simply because the ordinary Executive Officer could not give the necessary *time* to certain cases. The implication was that any EO could perform the task, given the time and that the swo was simply organisationally expedient. It was conceded that certain personalities would be more suited than others. But this is no more than a common-sense management technique, of putting square pegs in square holes. The notion of particular skill and expertise to be acquired was shunned since this would undoubtedly have raised problems of status in the powerful 'staff side'—the civil service trade unions whose influence on issues of this kind is considerable. In any case such notions go against the cherished belief in 'interchangeability' of civil servants. There have been—and still are—powerful arguments against specialisation that would limit mobility within the service. This is well illustrated by the dilemma of the swos. Acceptance of the view that their task requires similar, if not identical, skills to those of a social worker would logically lead to acceptance that they should be trained in the same way. But unless a separate professional career structure is envisaged, such swos, as civil servants, must expect on promotion to move on to other tasks. Therefore there is reluctance to invest too much money and time on training. Thus two obstacles can be seen to appropriate specialisation by skill rather than task: first, the problems of upgrading such specialisation within the existing structures; secondly, the diminished mobility that might result. This is not, of course, to imply that some specialisation by task is not useful, as for example in the case of Special Investigators who are required to investigate suspected abuse. It is simply to point out that the definition of specialisation is, at present, in certain ways somewhat confused, particularly with reference to those cases where the tasks to be performed are complex because they involve the interaction of financial, social and psychological factors.

There are four main kinds of specialist within the Supplementary Benefits administration. They are: Special Welfare Officers; Liable Relative Officers; Special Investigators; and Unemployment Review Officers. All swos, sis and most uros work from Regional offices. One region is exceptional in placing all uros within local offices, some of whom are part-time. In Scotland, the uros, although controlled from a central office, are based upon groups of local offices, lros are based in local offices. These may be full or part-time specialisations, according to the needs of the local office.

These specialists have considerable relevance to all the issues to be discussed in depth later in this book. Discussion here will therefore be confined to a factual description of their functions and an introduction to some of the issues arising from their role.

Special Welfare Officers

There are currently forty-seven swos in post. The cases are referred to swos by local offices and each swo covers a number of local offices. It will be obvious from the small numbers in relation to the total (about 420) of local offices that the coverage is scanty and that if the service were to be spread evenly, it would be very thin. In fact, it is recognised that some concentration of effort in certain areas is inevitable and not all local offices are covered by the service. The cases referred to swos fall into five main categories:

1. Inability or unwillingness to manage money—for example, rent arrears or other debts; repeated requests for exceptional needs payments.
2. Neglect of home, children, or self.
3. Difficulty in reduced circumstances—for example, newly-widowed or deserted women on lower incomes.
4. Difficulty in making satisfactory arrangements for the care of sick persons or invalids.
5. Difficulty in finding training, occupation, or normal employment for a disabled or handicapped person.

The overwhelming majority of referrals are of people in different kinds of financial difficulty—which is only to be expected and gives this social work its distinctive focus. A high proportion are suffering from some form of mental disorder. The swo carries a caseload of between twenty and forty. He is expected to liaise with the local social services, to avoid overlap and to refer wherever possible to the usual social work services. He is not a part of the local office team and is not at present part of a social work structure within a Regional office. Referral is at the discretion of the local office, which means that there are considerable variations in the extent to which the swo is used. The majority of the referrals are those in which a general anxiety, not always very clearly focused or understood, exists in the local office about the welfare of a claimant, the problem often manifesting itself in excessive demands on local office staff. As has been said earlier, the functions performed by the swo are essentially those of social work and the problems for the swo working in this organisation do not, as with some others, turn so much on role tension as on isolation and, to some extent, alienation from the mainstream of the work. They do not have the support of a professional reference group and in the writer's experience have very little contact with other social workers. Thus their situation is lonelier than that of others who may work alone within organisations not geared to social work but have a clear professional identity and frame of reference.

Liable Relative Officers
The title gives an indication of the job, which derives from the sections of the Social Security Act dealing with the liability of relatives. The LRO is primarily responsible for ensuring that men liable to maintain their wives and dependents do so, a duty placed upon the SBC by the Act. To this end, a large proportion of time is spent on administration—contact with magistrates courts, solicitors and local offices in other areas. Most LROs do little home visiting. However they have one responsibility which is of considerable interest to social workers—namely, the interviewing of women who come to the office to claim for the first time or to renew their claim. The majority of such women are either separated wives or have illegitimate children. In the case of the former, the woman caller is often in immediate need and calls at a point of crisis. (By the time a marital separation is formalised, an order book will usually be in payment, which will obviate the need to call at the office.) This means that a proportion, at any rate, are likely to be in distress. On the other hand, there are a proportion of women who allege desertion as a means of claiming benefit when in fact they are in contact with their husbands. The LRO is usually the officer to interview such women, and must inquire closely into the circumstances to ensure that the husband contributes what he can afford to the support of his family and that the claim is an honest one.

It is, incidentally, argued by some LROs that speedy action to contact the husbands in such cases is frequently more productive than if there is delay. There is the further problem that it is seldom possible to get a husband to pay arrears as well as current maintenance and the LRO is conscious of the responsibility to conserve public funds. They see this as a justification for asking these questions at an early stage. Similarly, in the case of the unmarried mother, the LRO is instructed to inquire into the paternity of the child and to encourage the mother to take out an affiliation order—this being to her advantage later if she ceases to claim benefit, as well as to the immediate advantage of the SBC. Questions of an intimate kind may on occasions be asked to establish whether there is likely to be a case for an affiliation order. Such interviews are conducted according to fairly precise instructions to protect both officer and claimant.

It will be obvious to the reader in this bare description that there is a potential tension between the role of the LRO and the general responsibility to have regard to the welfare of claimants. The fact that the LRO is thus firmly styled gives a clear indication of his primary focus. It is easy to see how such interviews, even if conducted with care and sensitivity by the officer, may be perceived as inappropriate or impertinent or as implying dishonesty on the part of the claimant. If they are not well conducted, these feelings are likely to be heightened. Furthermore, local office conditions are ideal for the purpose. Although a private interviewing room in local offices is a standard requirement, accommodation problems are such that this is not yet possible everywhere. However, it is officially recommended that 'sensitive' interviews should be conducted in private wherever possible.

In the opinion of the writer, the role of the specialist LRO is one that gives rise to greater problems in relation to welfare than any other. The foregoing illustrates the importance of understanding such problems in terms of role definition.

Special Investigators

There are at present 284 Special Investigators, who have been described by the SBC[1] as:

'Ordinary members of the staff of the Department who conduct enquiries . . . which any visiting office of the Department could conduct but which it is more sensible for selected staff rather than

[1] See Chapter 6 for a detailed discussion of the difficulties in which the cohabitation rule places Special Investigators and other officials. *Cohabitation*, SBC report to the Secretary of State for Social Services, HMSO, 1971.

local office staff to undertake because of their complex and time-consuming nature. They are specially selected only in the sense that some officers are clearly unsuitable, for example, because of inexperience or by temperament, for a job involving at least embarrassment and at worst a risk of physical violence.'

The Commission describes their job as 'to obtain evidence which will confirm or deny the information by claimants, in those cases where there is *prima facie* reason to doubt its accuracy'. Such inquiries may be in relation to three forms of suspected abuse; undisclosed earnings, fictitious or collusive desertion and undeclared cohabitation, all of which are to be discussed later in this book. There is no doubt that to most social workers such work is inherently distasteful and, however well it is carried out, is bound to be considered, on occasion, offensive by those of whom inquiries are made. 'It is unfortunate that, in the process, some people innocent of any desire to deceive the Commission will suffer the indignity of having their statements checked.' The Commission defend the use of SIS against those who argue 'that evidence obtained in this way would not stand up in a court of law'. This shows, they claim, 'a fundamental misunderstanding of the object of special enquiries . . . They are not intended to be automatically a preliminary to a prosecution . . . They are intended to discover facts on which to make a judgement about the case as a whole.' They point out that this may work in the claimants' favour—for example, by an allowance being increased.

Discussion of the use of the SIS takes us to the root of the tension between welfare and the protection of public funds—a tension which is the focus of much of this book. In this context, however, in which we are concerned simply to examine work roles, the following points should be made. First, if attempts are to be made to control abuse, someone has to do it. Who should that be? In some countries, in which means-tested benefits are not separate from social work, this is a job done by social workers, who inevitably dislike it intensely. The SI is, as emphasised by the Commission, an ordinary Executive Officer who has come from, and may well return to, ordinary duties. Distasteful as the job may be and allowing for the possibility that some SIS may act overzealously or unwisely, it is important that social workers should not stereotype such men as the private gestapo of the SBC. In the writer's opinion, there are considerable advantages in having a specialised team to investigate abuse. It may in fact work to protect claimants from the clouds of undispelled suspicion that sometimes hang over them when local office staff are worried about exploitation of the scheme and are too busy to investigate it further. Furthermore, the mere fact of having to refer a case to a SI sharpens the observations of the local office who must think out the basis of their suspicions, although the processes of such investigation are bound to be disturbing and distasteful to the claimant. Paradoxically, the greater use of SIS than at present might be, in the long term, of benefit to claimants generally, For, as will be considered later, with fatherless families particularly, harm may be done by an atmosphere within an office of anxious distrust about the honesty of claimants. Furthermore, the role of the SI is less ambiguous than some—for example, the Unemployment Review Officer, to be discussed next. He is required to be a detective and there is something reassuring in such a straightforward job definition; there are, nevertheless, obvious dangers. First, the SI has, by the nature of the task, considerable discretion in the way he does his work. Instructions too precisely detailed would hamper him unduly in investigations, the course of which cannot be predicted. In view of this and of the type of claimant he will sometimes be investigating, his selection and training become of great importance if the specialism is not to fall into ill-repute. Secondly, the question of welfare liaison is crucial. In a number of cases where dishonesty is established beyond reasonable doubt and the allowances are withdrawn, there are pressing financial problems as, for example, where a woman has claimed benefit as a deserted wife in desperation because her husband returns home erratically and does not support her adequately. There is little doubt that the SI has, in the past, seen his task as beginning and ending with the investigation and that referral back to the local office for action in relation to welfare has not always been made when it would have been appropriate. In this sense, the job definition has been over-simplified and exemplifies the danger that the dishonest will not be deemed deserving of 'welfare'.

Unemployment Review Officers

There are at present 120 posts for UROs—the numbers were doubled in 1970. The UROs have a responsibility to check the cases of unemployed claimants receiving supplementary benefit and, where appropriate, to take steps to encourage men back to work. The work is, of course, much affected by the employment position in a particular locality and the URO is sometimes limited in exercising his functions in areas of high unemployment.

The URO examines the case-papers of unemployed men and is

instructed not to interview certain categories: namely, men over 55 years, or in some areas over 60, depending on the local employment situation, and those with handicaps that seriously limit the type of work suitable for them. He will then request the men who remain to come to the office for an interview. At this stage a substantial number who do not come for interview go off the books and are thus presumed to have returned to work. With those who come for interview, the URO's task is clear, to get them back to work if, on interview, it appears possible to do so. But the means by which this is to be done are, of course, extremely varied. It could hardly be otherwise given the different attitudes, personalities and situations of the claimants concerned. The techniques employed, however, are not always related to an objective appraisal of the temperament and needs of a particular claimant; there may be occasions when it is the personality of the officer rather than that of the claimant which is the decisive factor. It is clear that UROs vary considerably in, to put it bluntly, the use of 'stick or carrot' techniques. Nor is it certain which gives better results in which cases—a matter that is currently the subject of research.[1] The limitations of the role, as at present structured, are, however, obvious. UROs have been instructed to make home visits and see the wife when the domestic situation was an important factor. However the URO, until recently, has paid few home visits, believing that the claimant would be more impressed by the seriousness of a request to visit the office. This may well be true in a number of cases. But it is clear that, in more complex situations, a follow-up visit to a family might be indispensable to the understanding, leave alone the treatment of the problem. There are signs that such visiting is now more common than it used to be, possibly as a result of the training now being given. Secondly—and most important from the point of view of welfare— is the fact that his success has been largely thought of as 'getting men off the books'. Recently, Headquarters has been at pains to stress that URO's work should not be judged by statistics alone, either in terms of numbers interviewed or numbers who go off the books. But the absence of other established criteria of success and the deeply entrenched view of the job in these terms at field level makes it difficult to effect change quickly. It is argued that for many men getting a job 'is the best welfare'. This argument is, in the writer's opinion, not to be cynically dismissed although one may question the extent to which, in this matter as in some other aspects of Supplementary Benefits administration, processes of rationalisation are at work to

[1] See Appendix II.

justify an activity initially prompted by a different concern, arising from the Social Security Act itself which laid a duty on the SBC to ensure that people did not claim supplementary benefit if they could maintain themselves. The URO is instructed to explore the cause of an individual's unemployment and then to do what he can to help with difficulties. He can always consider whether registration for work is appropriate at all. Nonetheless there are still cases in which social workers believe the assumption that the man should work is unreal or even unjustifiable. There are cases, for example, in which the low wages a man can command linked to the particular needs of his family may make it of no advantage economically and positively disadvantageous socially for him to work. As it stands, this is a possibility the URO cannot officially consider—which is not to say he may not do so unofficially, thus creating a certain role conflict. In fact, the URO, of all specialisations, sits firmly impaled on the horns of the now familiar, but nonetheless spikey, dilemma. His job was created to prevent abuse of the scheme, but the old NAB, and now the SBC have long realised that a fair proportion of the so-called 'work shy' have a variety of disabling psychological and social problems. The URO is neither selected nor trained to be a social worker. Yet as his work develops the relevance of some of these skills has begun to be considered.

Thus it can be seen that the specialisations discussed above are on a continuum in so far as 'welfare' and 'the protection of public funds are concerned. At one end, there is the SWO, reasonably comfortable in a role predominantly focused on welfare, although not free from tension in relation to the organisation as a whole. At the other end, there is the SI, again reasonably comfortable in a role which is essentially that of a detective, less likely to feel any sense of conflict and because of this at times an unwitting barrier to the official concern of the SBC for the welfare of its claimants. In the middle, are the LROs and UROs of whom, it is suggested, the latter are probably subject to the greatest ambiguity in the wider context of society's ambivalence towards unemployed men. However, the role definition of the LRO is, by reason of its deceptive simplicity, one in which potential dangers for the welfare of claimants are considerable.

CHAPTER 4

VOLUNTARY UNEMPLOYMENT I—
THE CLAIMANTS[1]

Definitions

The term 'voluntary unemployment' is loosely and somewhat con-
fusingly used within the SBC to cover both a subject and the attitudes
of mind of a range of claimants. The range of attitudes which it attempts
to describe varies from deliberately doing as little work as possible to
settling down on benefit without making any particular effort to find
work. The subject, however, is much wider, being concerned with
identifying such people and distinguishing them from those whose
unemployment is due either to the economic situation or to personal
handicaps of one kind or another, or to both, devising appropriate
procedures, and applying such sanctions, if any, as may be appropriate
in the individual case. Some sanctions are prescribed by statute,[2]
others are operated by the exercise of the Commission's discretion.
An underlying assumption is that some people, in greater or lesser
degree, have an attitude of wilful refusal. Official instructions now
limit this term to unemployment for which it is believed the claimant
is responsible through industrial misconduct, voluntarily leaving
employment or refusal of suitable employment 'without good cause'
and this may fairly be read as also covering unemployment which is
the result of not seeking suitable work known to be available.

Behind such an assumption, which necessitates forms of administrative action, is the judgement that the individual in question is capable
of modifying his behaviour—otherwise it would be 'involuntary'.
As every social worker knows, debates about freewill and determination
are of no help in considering particular cases. This discussion, while
using the term from time to time, is only concerned to throw light
upon the factors associated with the problem of men who do not work
or work most irregularly when it seems that there are jobs available.
However, it must be stressed that, even in areas of high employment,

---

[1] This chapter deals only with men. The problem in relation to women is quite insignificant numerically and nearly always related to some form of mental disorder or
acute personality disturbance.

[2] For example, see Section 1 (2) of the Social Security Act, 1971.

suitable jobs for the individuals concerned may not be available. For the men we are to consider are always 'marginal' in the employment market.

The Significance of the Problem[1]

It is generally agreed that the number of such men is quite small in relation to the total number of unemployed. They stand out more clearly at times of full employment. At the time of writing, rising unemployment serves to 'blur the edges' between those who are believed to seek work genuinely and those who are not. If the numbers are so small, why does the subject merit consideration at length? Why do all social security schemes in every country give attention to the problem and seek to evolve techniques of controlling it? The answer lies in the profound emotional significance of work in Western societies and in the uncertainty that exists not so much about the current extent of the problem as in 'the fear of contagion'. That is to say, those who administer the scheme are concerned not only with a particular case but with the effects that their handling of particular cases may have on a wider group of potential or actual recipients of supplementary benefits. This, of course, cannot be precisely determined although attempts to estimate it in terms of trends over a period of time could be made if policies were varied. Yet such estimates will not establish a direct link between cause and effect because there will be other intervening variables. Thus it must be conceded that the extent to which social security policy, in terms of allowances paid to, and treatment of, unemployed men, affects the willingness of 'the average man' to work is and will remain largely a matter of opinion rather than of fact, even if more sophisticated research techniques than exist at present are evolved. However this makes the argument all the stronger for examination in depth and detail of what can be learnt about the problem. For it is by the treatment of unemployed men that the sincerity of Supplementary Benefits welfare policy may be judged. Formal policies in relation to unemployment and their application in practice demonstrate more clearly than in any other sphere of Supplementary Benefits administration the tension between the need to protect public funds and the need to have regard to individual welfare. This is an inevitable tension but one which it is difficult to keep properly balanced, and in the absence of concrete knowledge the administration is more vulnerable to pressure. The right and the obligation to work has been a very important aspect of social philo-

[1] See also Appendix I.

sophy in western-type societies. This is an underlying theme in the following discussion since administrative processes in the public service are to some extent a reflection of basic attitudes in a given society at a point in time. In the context of a debate about 'voluntary unemployment' it is important to consider the extent to which the SBC can, does or should mirror in its policies the variety in public opinion. It is not the intention here to examine the underlying assumptions of 'a work-orientated society'. In contrast to the dedication of a pioneering society such as Israel (in which unemployment benefit has only very recently become a part of the social security provision) or of the USA,[1] Great Britain appears somewhat less passionate on this issue. Certainly the measures taken to control the problem are not as drastic as in many other countries. Reactions against the 'Protestant ethic' which has so strongly emphasised the moral value of work for the individual can be detected in the younger generation both here and in other countries, including the USA. It is too early to say whether this is limited to particular and exceptional groups or whether their influence will spread. Furthermore, the effects of rising unemployment among a generation, many of whom, unlike their fathers, had never before experienced problems in getting work when they wished, have yet to be gauged. Such experiences might reinforce the importance of work to groups of young people who might otherwise have been influenced by the attitudes of some of their peers. This is, of course, highly speculative. It is, however, a matter of fact that among the unemployed clientele of the SBC there are a certain number of young people who drift around the country, following each other to certain areas such as seaside resorts in the summer, working a little and claiming a little as the fancy takes them. They do not subscribe to the idea of obligation to work. Their numbers are not large and they may indeed be the modern equivalent of the 'sturdy beggar', present in all societies at all times. Alternatively, they may reflect the beginning of certain trends against the value systems of our society in which work is one important element. It is easy to confuse moral values and psychological benefits in this matter. Many, especially the medical profession, emphasise the psychological importance of work, as witnessed by the significance which is attached to it in physical and mental rehabilitation. As a background to the following discussion it should be borne in mind that whatever reservations there may be in individual cases concerning the appropriateness of employment as a psychological goal there is a

[1] In some states of the USA unemployed men and women are not eligible for public assistance.

F

deeply rooted belief in our society that, to put it simply, 'work is good for you'. Such a belief is open to challenge but must not be lightly dismissed in an appraisal of administrative policy.

However, there is no doubt that much of public concern is focused upon the more specific issue—that public funds should not be used to support those who are capable of work. Social workers need to be reminded of this since in their proper preoccupation with the way individuals are treated these pressures on the Supplementary Benefits administration, typified by letters to the press and questions in the House of Commons, tend to be overlooked. It would be extremely naive to suppose that forms of external constraint or incentive are not relevant for us all in the will to work. It is equally naive to suppose that this is all that is relevant in the understanding of those who do or do not work. What follows is an attempt to outline some of the factors that may be important in understanding 'the voluntarily unemployed'.

The Statutory Responsibilities of the SBC

Before doing so, the statutory responsibilities of the SBC must be clarified. These are set out in the Supplementary Benefits Handbook[1] as follows:

'Under the Act, a man is liable to maintain his wife and children: a woman is liable to maintain her husband and her children ... And every person, man or woman, is liable to maintain himself. Thus it follows that unless there are good reasons why a person should not be in work, the Commission cannot be expected to pay a Supplementary allowance indefinitely.

Payment of an allowance to an able-bodied man is intended to meet his needs and those of his dependents while he cannot do so himself. Where it appears that a person claiming or in receipt of a supplementary allowance who is not receiving unemployment benefit refuses or neglects to maintain himself or his dependents by working, receipt of benefit can be made conditional upon his attendance at a re-establishment centre ... an industrial rehabilitation unit or a training centre. Where refusal or neglect is persistent, he may be prosecuted. In circumstances where unemployment benefit, if in payment, would be suspended or disallowed ... *and* it is known that there is a particular job, open to the claimant and suitable for him, a supplementary allowance may be refused or summarily stopped. Such action is not taken in the case of a registered disabled

[1] The Supplementary Benefits Handbook, Paras 162, 166, 167.

person or anyone with a serious physical or mental disability or where there are dependents, especially children, who would suffer hardship.

In the general run of cases, however, voluntary unemployment is controlled by practical methods, developed in the light of the Commission's duty to "exercise its functions in such manner as shall best promote the welfare of persons affected by the exercise thereof".'

Such a statement makes clear the areas of judgement and discretion in this aspect of the Commission's activities, stemming from the basic question of a man's fitness, mental or physical to work, of his social circumstances and of employment opportunities. At various levels in the organisation decisions to suspend or disallow benefit, to make it conditional upon various forms of training, and to prosecute have to be taken. The 'practical methods' to control voluntary employment have to be reconciled with 'welfare'. Behind such bald comments lies an extremely delicate area of administration. Before considering the way these issues are, or should be handled, the complexity of the human problems behind the administrative process needs to be fully considered.

The man we seek to understand is an individual, a member of a family, and of a wider social group, including at some stage or other, a work group. These will be considered in turn in relation to his unemployment but the question of economic incentive, so frequently stressed as crucial, will be discussed first.

Economic Incentives

As has already been indicated, no-one could be so ingenuous as to suppose that economic incentive for work is unimportant. It is clear that this is, however, closely related to the motivation of particular individuals. There is no clear-cut point at which a comparison of wages with Supplementary Benefits scales can lead us to say with confidence that the incentive for that particular individual to work had been eliminated. Bakke,[1] whose penetrating analysis in 'The Unemployed Man' of the issues arising from the introduction of unemployment benefit has as much relevance today as then, wrote: 'It is impossible to draw a line and say "On this side there are those who are likely to attempt to live on the state and on the other side are those who are likely not to do so". The causes which lead to malingering are complicated circumstances.'

[1] E. Bakke, 'The Unemployed Man: A social Study', in R. A. Nisbet (ed.), 1933.

Bakke goes on to consider a variety of circumstances of which the 'scale of wages' is one. The fact is that very large numbers of the population are in low-paid and uncongenial employment and show no inclination to give it up. Of course it is impossible to guess how many would thankfully relinquish it if social security benefits came without questions asked. There has been a reaction against a sentimentalised view of the intrinsic satisfactions of work, especially if it comes from those whose experience of work bears little relation to the hard, monotonous and distasteful work that is the lot of many. It is equally clear that the incentive of wages much higher than social security benefits is bound to be powerful. It is extremely difficult to obtain reliable data that would clarify the extent to which men were rationally deterred from working for this reason. Nevertheless, as a rough generalisation, for those receiving supplementary benefits who would in employment command low wages the economic disincentive to work probably becomes strongest for a man with four or more children.[1] The basic entitlement at the 1971 scale rates (excluding rent or exceptional circumstance allowances) for one child of eleven years and four younger, is £18.10 per week. This compares favourably with the net earnings, without overtime, of an unskilled worker.

The Wage Stop

It is in such situations that the 'wage stop' provisions become relevant. The case for it has been argued by the SBC in their paper.[2] It is to be noted that the Commission specifically deny that the purpose of the wage stop provision is to provide an incentive to get work. 'The principle is that it would be unfair to the man who was working but earning less than the supplementary benefits level if his counterpart who was unemployed received a higher income'. Thus the wage stop is intended to leave the unemployed claimant neither better nor worse off than he would be when working.[3] Whatever the principle, however, it is obvious that, for some claimants, full supplementary benefit allowances which were not related to earning power would act as a disincentive to work. Such may sometimes be the situation in cases in which the wage stop is not applied, or is discontinued, as for example when a man has been ill for more than three months or where a man, although not certified as incapable of work, has been unemployed for

---

[1] See Lafitte in *Socially Deprived Families*, (Ed.) Holman, Bedford Square Press, London, 1970.

[2] *The Administration of the Wage Stop*, HMSO, 1967.

[3] See 'The Supplementary Benefit Handbook', Para. 69.

a long time and is seriously handicapped. It is frequently argued that payment of a supplementary allowance below the minimum subsistence levels on which supplementary benefit is calculated is morally wrong. This is irrefutable. It leads, however, to a consideration of the wage structure of the country and of alternative methods of family support (for example, of family allowances, negative income tax and so on) rather than to an indictment of the wage stop *per se*. Certainly if the wage stop were removed the individual claimant would be in a genuine moral dilemma as to whether he should work or allow his family the benefit of a higher standard of living. The introduction of the Family Income Supplement is, in principle, an important innovation that has a bearing on this problem. Of course, much depends in practice on its scope and there are cogent arguments against a reintroduction of a latter day 'Speenhamland system' because of the encouragement it may provide to keep wages low. However, it must affect the application of the wage stop since there are families whose low earning power is supplemented by the Family Income Supplement and whose allowances, therefore, in times of unemployment are calculated in terms of wages plus Family Income Supplement rather than by wages alone. However, the effects on work incentives are at present uncertain.

In a written parliamentary answer in December 1971, it was stated that 'the number of claimants whose supplementary benefit was reduced under the wage stop provisions fell from about 18,000 to just under 4,000 when the Family Income Supplement was introduced at the beginning of August. But for the introduction of Family Income Supplement the pre-August figure would have risen very considerably when supplementary benefit scale rates were increased in September 1971; in fact the number of persons affected by the wage stop in November 1971 was 20,838.[1]

Even for the wage-stopped claimant, there may be some financial incentive or disincentive to work. In theory he should receive the same as he would in employment. In fact, this is difficult to calculate with precision and there are frequently cases in which he finds himself marginally better or worse off. In such cases other aspects of the situation will probably determine his willingness to seek employment.

Discussion of economic incentives has tended to be over simplified by those who may think of themselves as opposing factions. There are those—including some officials—who view the claimant with cynicism and see his reluctance to work as a sign that he is comfortable

[1] Hansard, Vol. 828, No. 37, p. 5.

in his way of life, even when standards are low. Social workers, on the other hand, point to poverty, to allowances that may on occasion be below subsistence level and they therefore doubt the existence of a financial disincentive to work. (Alternatively, they may on occasion question whether finding work is a desirable object at all, given the family circumstances.) Either argument may reflect aspects of the truth in certain cases: both, if taken in isolation, do less than justice to the complexity of people's material and social problems and the interaction between them.

Social and Psychological Factors

Having considered the matter of economic incentives, we turn now to examine those social and psychological factors that are of importance in the understanding of the problem. What follows arises from the writer's investigation of the problem as Social Work Adviser and the suggestions put forward are based upon scrutiny of many case-papers, discussions with many officials at various levels in the organisation and on visits to unemployed claimants. No validity for the observations can be claimed as in carefully conducted research. Furthermore, the frames of reference upon which one draws to understand any problem inevitably affect the observations themselves as well as the conclusions drawn from them. Such qualifications, together with the writer's conviction that the problem is a crucial one in welfare policy led to proposals for research, which is now under way, sponsored by the Department of Health and Social Security. Appendices I and II outline this research, the conclusions of which are not available at the time of writing.

Motivation for work may be connected with, but cannot often be said with certainty to be causally related to, varieties of personal and social disability. In other words, one can always point to the man who has overcome a variety of difficulties in order to work—physical, mental, familial. The fact that one frequently sees such difficulties among the so-called 'voluntarily unemployed' can rarely therefore be a total explanation. It is possible, however, to think in terms of a 'balance of probabilities'; that is to say, given the attitudes, personality and abilities of a certain individual, associated problems may load the dice against certain men getting work.

Attitudes to Work

Consideration of social attitudes to work must also take into account the occupational expectations of some men. If they have particular skills they will not, at any rate in the early stages, be subject to the same pressure as the unskilled to take any available employment. However, that is not the end of the story. The research in progress hopes to throw light on the number of unskilled unemployed men who appear to be dissatisfied with the type of work they can get. The dissatisfaction may or may not be related to earnings. Initial impressions suggest that this problem may not be insignificant among younger men; if the findings bear this out, some interesting issues concerning the relationship between intellectual ability, educational attainment and occupational opportunity may be raised. However, among the so-called 'voluntarily unemployed' there are probably more whose attitudes to work derive not from particular occupational expectations but from the values of their particular subculture. Experienced officials know all too well that there are certain men whose irregular or casual employment, supplemented by supplementary benefits, is as normal a way of life as the war waged by the middle classes against the Tax Inspector. Their battles to outwit officialdom are part and parcel of a general attitude to a society to whose standards they do not subscribe and may be associated with delinquency. Not infrequently, such men have forms of lucrative employment 'on the side' and the supplementary allowance which they claim is a useful addition to their income. They know that they are taking a risk and expect to discontinue their claim from time to time 'when the heat is on'. When the Unemployment Review Officers visit a local office, a substantial proportion of the men they call go off the books before the interview. It is generally assumed that the majority of these either get jobs or decide to live on what they have in fact been earning. Such an assumption, however, cannot go unquestioned without further study. We do not, for example, know how far these 'successes' are in fact only a reflection of the normal turnover of unemployed men. Nor do we know how many 'innocent' people are frightened away. There are many unanswered questions about such a group which are of intrinsic interest to the social scientist and the social worker and which have implications for the Supplementary Benefits administration. Not least among these is the notion of the 'happy delinquent', cheerfully plying his trade, pitting his wits against authority which is therefore absolved from any responsibility except 'to catch the villain'. Close scrutiny of so-called delinquent subcultures has often revealed patterns of family disturbance and distress, and of mental disorder. However, from the point of view of the Supplementary Benefits administration, the existence of such a group seems to imply a need for differential treatment between them and those claimants whose individual and interpersonal difficulties are of relevance to their unemployment. The problem for the administration is to spot the difference and to avoid a climate of suspicion among officials that would cloud judgement in individual cases.

'Inadequacy'

This is not made easier by the fact that there is no clear-cut distinction between 'the villains' and the 'unfortunates'. A word frequently used in this context in Supplementary Benefit records, as in social work, is 'inadequate'. It is vague and frequently perjorative. It attempts to describe those who are neither successfully delinquent not mentally disordered but who make up a fair proportion of 'the voluntarily unemployed'. It is, of course, not uncommon for such men to be on the fringes of the delinquent subculture. When the term is analysed further in relation to particular individuals one finds it refers to an amalgam of characteristics—physical, mental and emotional—present in varying degree although it is essentially a term descriptive of poor social functioning. Such descriptions have to be related to the employment that may be available for the individual in question. It is the impression of the writer that a significant proportion of those whose presenting behaviour suggests their unemployment may be 'voluntary' are of poor physique and prone to minor illness and injury. Their capacity to undertake heavy labouring work may be limited and they do not commend themselves to prospective employers when they present themselves. Furthermore, their chances of obtaining such work steadily diminish with age. They may also be markedly below average in intellectual capacity.[1] This is a matter of considerable concern in view of trends towards automation and a diminishing market for unskilled labour. Thus poor physical and mental equipment may in itself produce a situation in which, even in areas of high employment, 'our man' is at a grave disadvantage in the labour market. Intellectual inadequacy may shade off into subnormality. Its detection by officials is not always a simple matter, especially when the claimant has verbal facility. A number who fail in employment, with consequent discouragement, may be quite severely subnormal. Alternatively, the claimant may be educationally inadequate whatever his intellectual potential.

'Emotional inadequacy' is yet more difficult to define with precision and in this context is associated with weak motivation to work,

[1] It is hoped that the research in progress will throw further light on this.

proneness to becoming discouraged, difficulty in planning purposefully —a range of characteristics with which social workers are all too familiar. For the Supplementary Benefits official this nebulous type of description poses problems. Administrative policy requires judgements as to whether men are capable of work and officials long for these judgements to be clear-cut and based, for example, on a diagnosis of physical or mental incapacity. Although, as will be shown later, such a diagnosis does not in fact dispose of the question of work motivation, it at least offers a label to which the administrative system can respond. 'The inadequate' offers no such clear-cut description, for one must ask: inadequate relative to what, how inadequate and so on. It requires a judgement of social functioning, a weighing-up of probabilities in relation to particular individuals. It is rare for psychiatrists who examine such men for the Commission to commit themselves to the view that they are 'unfit for work' since they are often not psychiatrically ill in the conventional sense. Yet it is beyond doubt that a substantial proportion of the 'voluntarily unemployed' do fall into this category, vague though it may be. Thus in any scheme that attempts to combine firmness with humanity the assessment and treatment of such individuals as *individuals*, not as categories, is crucial.

Mental Illness

There are a certain number of unemployed claimants who suffer from mental illness with clear-cut clinical symptoms. When this is perceived by officials and psychiatric referral can be made they may no longer present an administrative problem. A medical certificate is usually— as far as the SBC is concerned—the end of the matter. Of course, this does not mean the individual concerned may not need ongoing help in relation to employment, as with other aspects of his social situation, for a number of the mentally disordered are capable of work in sheltered or carefully selected situations. (Some such men will find their way onto the books of the Department of Employment and Productivity's Disablement Resettlement Officer. This affords yet another illustration of the way in which organisational and administrative fragmentation affects treatment of individuals. Social workers will be familiar with this, for example in the field of child welfare in which separate provisions have existed for the so-called 'deprived', 'delinquent', and 'maladjusted' child.) But a medical diagnosis can take these men off the list of those who are considered to be potentially 'voluntarily unemployed'.

The problems for the Supplementary Benefits administration, therefore, are twofold: first, how to ensure that such mental illness is
detected and second, how to make balanced judgements in those
spheres of mental disorder that are less precisely defined in psychiatric
terms—notably in the matter of psychopathy and of physical symptoms
of emotional disorder. Both questions have important implications
for the selection, organisation and training of Supplementary Benefits
staff.

A sufficient skill in observation to remark upon the possibility of
mental illness, and therefore to refer, cannot be taken for granted in
the Supplementary Benefits official. The observations social workers
and others in related fields make about appearances and behaviour as
a matter of course result from their primary motivation to understand
such difficulties, reinforced by their training. Furthermore, their
work affords them greater opportunity to observe. (Friday afternoon
at the counter is not a time or a situation in which perception of
individuals is heightened.) The difficulties are increased in those forms
of mental disorder that are concealed or those that attract less attention
because the symptoms are nearer to normal behaviour. In the case of
the former, paranoid illnesses are the most likely to baffle the official
(as any other layman), since it may take a considerable time before
delusions that may be central to a man's reluctance to take employment are revealed. Among the latter, depressive illnesses present
particular difficulties because the officials may be unable to distinguish
between these and what he may term 'idleness'. This is sometimes
illustrated by irritable references in records to visits paid in mid-
morning—'Claimant still in bed'. In a proportion (by no means all)
of such cases, there will be a depressive illness. In general, to know
how seriously to take symptoms that are an extension and exaggeration
of feelings, such as depression and anxiety—which most of us experience consciously—is extremely hard for the lay official. A further
difficulty is that even if mental disorder is suspected, it may not be
possible to persuade the claimant to accept referral and it may not be
appropriate to make a referral against his wishes. In such cases there
can be no escape from the exercise of administrative discretion in
deciding whether to press the individual to take employment.

As has been mentioned, psychopathy and some kinds of physical
symptoms present particular problems in this respect. The 1959
Mental Health Act, which first brought the term 'psychopathy' into
legal use, offered the following definition: 'Psychopathic disorder
means a persistent disorder or disability of mind . . . which results in

abnormally aggressive or seriously irresponsible conduct on the part of the patient.' Thus the definition rests in part on a matter of degree—behaviour which is *abnormally* aggressive or *seriously* irresponsible. The term describes the behaviour of an individual towards others: a judgement as to the degree of disturbance must also involve an appreciation of the interactional factors (such as provocation) which may have led to such behaviour and of the differences in acceptable behaviour between different social groups and classes. There has been much dispute about the validity of the classification among lawyers and psychiatrists; moral judgements frequently lurk behind the term. Therefore officials have received little help and support from medical and psychiatric experts in relation to these claimants who are, however, particularly difficult to understand and to handle in relation to employment. They may be aggressive or full of glib promises that are never kept; they may take work but fall out quickly with foreman or mates and they are prone to impulsive behaviour, such as walking out on the job. They have difficulty in establishing and maintaining relationships so that the efforts of the well-intentioned to place them in employment will often fail.

Physical Symptons

Physical symptoms of emotional disorder also present considerable difficulties to the Supplementary Benefits administration and raise the question of a definition of 'malingering', a phrase which carries an implication that the illness is simulated and results in a calculated plan of work avoidance. It appears to the writer, on the basis of cases studied, that the number of claimants who consciously invent symptoms having no foundation in fact were probably few. Such a group may be described as malingerers, although using this somewhat loaded term does not dispose of the problem since a persistent pattern of this kind may in itself be indicative of a personality disorder. However, far more common are the men who exploit minor ailments. That is to say, there is some degree of bodily disturbance but it is used by one individual to avoid facing certain situations whereas another individual would overcome it. Physical illness is a respectable and acceptable excuse within certain limits. It is far easier for a man to say: 'I have the flu and so cannot work' than 'I am depressed and so cannot work'. However, *repeated* evasions of this sort rapidly incur censure and even less tolerance than outright mental illness. When such symptoms are persistently offered, their very persistence in the face of moral outrage and censure on the part of 'authority'—be it doctors, officials or employers—suggests the importance of looking behind the symptoms to the underlying reasons, for example, a man's domestic or working relationship.

A third group whose problems centre on somatic functioning are those whose feelings, which give rise to the symptoms, are unconscious. Into this category fall those who believe themselves to have illnesses where none exist or who have produced a physical illness in which it is thought that psychological factors play an important part. This latter group will usually not represent a problem to the Department, since their illness, whatever its causation, is not in question. It is possible, however, that the former group might be mistaken for the 'malingerers' described above, at least until the intractable and painful nature of their anxieties has made it clear that some different factors were at work.

Such symptoms, springing as they do from sources of which the patient is unaware, are peculiarly difficult to treat and, if they affect a man's working capacity, the chances of improvement in that sphere are remote, whereas the man who 'exploits minor ailments' may feel less need to do so if he is helped to feel more confident. It is likely that of those claimants who present physical symptoms as a reason for working but who are not certified by the medical experts as unfit for not working but who are not certified by the medical experts as unfit poses the most awkward administrative problem. This is made the more complicated by inconsistency in the medical profession who vary considerably in their readiness to issue medical certificates and in their attitudes towards unemployed men.

Family Interaction

There are a number of other claimants, however, who cannot be described as mentally ill but whose interpersonal family difficulties are such that they do not work. It is of course dangerous to attempt a rigid distinction between those who are ill and those who are not. The distinctions are always somewhat arbitrary since 'illness' is a relative and not an absolute term and they may encourage a sharp division in administrative policy between 'sickness' and 'sinning'. However, in our present state of understanding, it seems inevitable that such distinctions will continue and their arbitrariness will have to be tolerated. Nevertheless, a deeper understanding of the effect a man's family and domestic circumstances may have upon his attitude towards employment may counterbalance this. The subtlety of the processes involved are rarely recognised within the SBC, which is hardly surprising since the development of knowledge in the field of family interaction is relatively new; social workers and psychiatrists have only recently begun to think in these terms.[1] This work has increasingly stressed that the behaviour of the family must be viewed as a total system in which the individuals affect, and are affected by, other family members to an extent hitherto not fully recognized. Thus there are some who believe that patterns of distorted or incomplete communications between members of a family play a part in producing mental illness in one of them—although the probability of constitutional factors is not denied. Others studying marital interaction have emphasised that one partner may encourage or even provoke behaviour in the other to express attitudes or feelings which the former cannot admit to openly. An over-simplified example is woman who is 'meek and mild, the down-trodden, good little woman' with the violent husband. She may derive some satisfaction from his aggression, not only to her but to others, while she watches from the sidelines. Recent work emphasises the subtlety and complexity of such interaction.

It will readily be seen how such theories—now current and prolifer-ting—may affect our view of the problem of voluntary unemployment. A not uncommon example is the single man, perhaps in his forties, living with his mother. Sometimes he is known to have been mentally ill but in other cases no illness has been diagnosed, yet he is clearly emotionally immature and excessively dependent on his mother. There may, of course, be circumstances that have created or exacerba-ted this dependency—such as the man's low intelligence or physical disability. But one must also be alive to the possibility that the mother plays her part in encouraging this dependency, sometimes by an unconscious technique of confusing and undermining her son's belief in his adequacy as a man. Nor can this always be readily observed. There are times when the maternal attitudes that have undermined the son are concealed behind a conscious wish to 'do the best' for him. In the marital relationship many factors may affect a man's attitude to work, some of which are discussed below. For officials, one of the most difficult aspects of this is that, in this most complex sphere of relationships, perhaps above all others, what people say—even if consciously believed at that moment—does not necessarily represent their true feelings or represents them only in part. Nor is it beyond possibility that a wife who is most 'cooperative' (to use the Depart-ment's word) about her husband's refusal to work and who criticises him to the officer, is joining with authority to turn him into the black

---

[1] See, for example, the works of Laing, Ackerman and the Institute of Marital Studies listed in Appendix III.

sheep, while she (unconsciously) projects herself as snow-white. If this pattern is reinforced by the authorities, the man may be driven further and further into his antisocial behaviour.

Family Problems

In drawing attention to these less obvious aspects of family problems the obvious must not be overlooked. There are, of course, families in which severe practical problems, such as the illness or absence of the wife, have a direct bearing on the huskand's unemployment. However, although it may occasionally raise administrative problems, which will be discussed in the next chapter, it is not as complicated from the point of view of *understanding* the claimant's apparent refusal to take work.

In the course of discussions with social workers and officers, certain patterns of individual behaviour and of marital and family interaction which bear on employment problems have been suggested. They are speculative and it is hoped that some assessment of their validity will be made in the course of the research which has been referred to. In the meantime, it may be of value to mention and to illustrate them briefly since they highlight the importance of the attempt to understand behaviour and interaction which does not fall under any established clinical headings.

The Family of Origin

A person's current attitudes to work derive in part from childhood learning and socialisation. Thus one would expect to find that some men had the childhood model of a father who did not work. There is ample evidence from case records to suggest that there are some families in which the patterns of unemployment or erratic employment are handed down from father to son. This may well be associated with forms of antisocial behaviour and must be understood in the context of social norms generally. We have little evidence about the work patterns of men whose fathers had, for reasons of domestic circumstances or personality traits, stayed at home to look after them. This is a matter on which concrete evidence would be of value since officials of the Supplementary Benefits administration express concern at the long-term effects on the children of 'a father who stays at home'. Examination of case records seemed to suggest that attitudes to work were not infrequently associated with a father-son relationship in which negative feelings predominated. In such cases, it might well be that the son's refusal to work was a reflection of his antagonism to his father, especially when the latter (as was not infrequent) had been a regular worker. A Probation Officer wrote:

'Mr A has never worked regularly since he left school . . . He hates his father whom he alleges was cruel to him as a child. He has resentful aggressive attitudes towards men . . . He loses jobs through quarrels with the foremen. He fought his father about going to work —it was a way of getting back at him.'

The Home Office research study, *Probationers in their Social Environment*,[1] has drawn attention to the relevance of probationers' relationships with their fathers to the success of their probation order. They also analyse the work records of the youths (between 17 and 21 years). Unfortunately for the purposes of this discussion, they do not correlate the 'father relationship' patterns with work records. However, from social work experience, it seems probable that, in a proportion of cases, poor relationships with fathers will have engendered a general distrust of and antagonism to authority which is likely to affect attitudes to work and to officials concerned with employment.

Men who want to be mother

The SBC is not infrequently confronted with problems of men whose wives have left them and who want to stay at home to look after the children. In such situations it is not the policy of the SBC to bring pressure to bear on the men unless satisfactory arrangements can be made for the care of the children, especially those under school age. (Formal policies are only half the story and there is little doubt that prejudice exists in the minds of officers about such situations, as will be discussed later.) Such arrangements may in some cases be extremely difficult or impossible to make and practical problems should not be underestimated in enthusiasm for psychological explanations. Nevertheless it has not escaped the observant official that some men appear to derive considerable satisfaction from this maternal role and it is not uncommon in these circumstances for the children to be better cared for than when the mother was at home. This is hardly surprising since we now acknowledge that the boundaries between masculinity and femininity are not rigid. Goldberg[2] has discussed the variety in 'marital fit' in which the balance of sexual identification between partners plays a crucial part. In recent years masculine and feminine roles have be-

[1] M. Davies, *Probationers in their Social Environment*, HMSO, 1969.
[2] E. Goldberg, 'The Normal Family—Myth and Reality' in *Social Work with Families*, (Ed.), E. Younghusband, Allen & Unwin, London, 1965.

come much more flexible, especially in relation to child-rearing and a young generation may find nothing strange in the 'maternal' role of a father. Here, however, the more conventional traditional attitudes within the s b c, linked perhaps to lack of knowledge about the importance of consistency in parental care, especially with children separated from their mothers, may lead to difficulties in practice, if not in official policy. Suspicions that a man is content to stay at home are aroused if he appears to be enjoying it too much! Such maternal aspirations are, of course, partly unconscious and very powerful. Sometimes they are a source of conflict and ambivalence. At other times they seem dominant. For the official it may be impossible to gauge the extent and reality of the practical difficulties in alternative care for the children put forward. The social worker, especially those formerly involved in child care, will readily acknowledge such drives but will usually take the view that they are in no way morally reprehensible and should be accepted for what they are, especially when the gains to the children of a stable home are obvious. However, we have little evidence as to the long-term psychological effects on the children of this shift from conventional roles.

The following—admittedly rather extreme—example shows how powerful this urge may be:

'Mr B is now 46, with seven children, between 2 and 14 years. He has been unemployed for many years; prosecution was considered but dropped following a suicide threat. The case record is liberally sprinkled with accounts of failed appointments with medical officers and psychiatrists. The wife deserted on several occasions, leaving the children. She left him finally and, at the last check, Mr B was at home "being mother".'

The interest of this example lies in the references throughout the records, culminating in the report below from the Manager, which points in the direction of the eventual outcome.

'The relations between husband and wife are poor. The man appears very aware of his importance at home and does much to impress all agencies with this. The mother is constantly denigrated by our claimant, possibly in an effort to compensate for the deficiencies of which he is well aware in his own role.'

The psychiatrist who eventually saw him reported:

'He at no time made any attempt to defend himself or to protest, save on one occasion when, saying that he knew he was locally regarded as a malingerer, pointed out *that he had never claimed maternity benefit'* (My italics).

The Inability to Separate

Among the so-called 'problem families', one not infrequently hears of couples who, despite violent quarrels and a family chaos of debt and dirt, stick together 'through thick and thin' and are to be seen everywhere together (including the Department's offices) with a collection of children in train. Commendable as this matrimonial solidarity may appear to be, it is inevitably associated with unemployment. The parents concerned are usually over-burdened with children, so that it is understandable that the woman needs her husband to share the family responsibilities. Looking more deeply at the problem, however, one can also see in the deprived and unstable family backgrounds from which they usually come the roots of the emotional need to cling together.[1] Through this very closeness and the intensity of the need which each has to be 'mothered' or 'fathered' by the other, there are bound to be tensions when needs clash or are not met.

A different pattern that may sometimes be observed is where the 'parenting' of one partner by the other is one-sided rather than mutual. Dora, the child-wife in Charles Dickens' *David Copperfield*, is an example of this and in this instance the man assumes a role which is, in a sense, both maternal and paternal. It is surprising that David Copperfield was not 'voluntarily unemployed'; had it not been for Betsy Trotwood, who mothered Dora, he might well have been.

"I am not blaming you, Dora. We have both a great deal to learn. I am trying to show you, my dear, that you must—you really must (I was resolved not to give this up) accustom yourself to look after Mary Anne (the maid). Likewise to act a little for yourself, and me."

"I wonder, I do, at your making such ungrateful speeches," sobbed Dora, "when you know that the other day, when you said you would like a little bit of fish, I went out myself, miles and miles, and ordered it, to surprise you."

"And it was very kind of you, my own darling," said I. "I felt it so much that I wouldn't on any account have even mentioned that you bought a salmon which was too much for two. Or that it cost one pound six—which was more than we can afford."

[1] See F. Philip, *Family Failure*, Faber, London, 1963.

G

"You enjoyed it very much," sobbed Dora. "And you said I was a mouse."

"And I'll say so again, my love," I returned, "A thousand times!"

'But I had wounded Dora's soft little heart, and she was not to be comforted. She was so pathetic in sobbing and bewailing, that I felt as if I had said I don't know what to hurt her. *I was obliged to hurry away; I was kept out late; and I felt all night such pangs of remorse as made me miserable. I had the conscience of an assassin, and was haunted by a vague sense of enormous wickedness*' (My italics).

Such extremes are fortunately rare but there are unemployed men who are kept at home by their wives because the degree of dependence on them is so great. In such cases it may be the man's inability to refuse his wife and his guilt at distressing her rather than any particular wish on his part to stay at home which is the crucial factor. One would expect to find the wife in poor health, or suffering from anxieties at being left alone in the house. The man will frequently fear for her safety or that she will leave him.

The other version of this marital dependency is the one in which—as we often hear—'the man is really the eldest child in the family'. In such cases the immaturity of the one is reinforced by the dominance of the other. The wives may be over-protective of their husbands, to the point of colluding with them in evading the strictures of authority. In this connection, it is interesting to note that, in a small official survey of men prosecuted for voluntary unemployment, there were twice as many 'husband younger' marriages as in the general population.[1]

Separated Couples

Mention must also be made of men separated from their wives. The financial difficulties that arise are frequently due to the man's inability to support two families. In some cases, however, the bitterness felt towards the wife is such that a man will deliberately give up jobs after orders have been made for attachment of earnings. Much more difficulty is experienced in getting men to pay for wives than for children, and the sense of grievance which some men have about orders to pay their wives is obviously in some instances justified, both in terms of their wives' current circumstances and in terms of the earlier matrimonial difficulties, in which both parties played their part.

Such are a few of the variations of marital interaction that are likely

[1] See Chapter 5.

to have a bearing on the problem of voluntary unemployment. It will be appreciated that, in matters of this kind, there are no absolute distinctions, no hard and fast lines between the patterns nor between those who manage or do not manage to work with such difficulties. Whether or not such difficulties are associated with unemployment will depend partly on the intensity of the problem and partly on other associated factors, such as large numbers of children and the relative inaccessibility of work, which tip the balance.

Patterns of Work

In attempting to understand the difficulties of those who present serious employment problems there is much to be gained by studying the patterns of a man's employment record, going back as far as possible. It is also useful, with younger men, to examine their school attendance records. And it is relevant to ask—'Did father work?' and 'do the other brothers work?' Where the pattern is long-standing and is one shared by close relations, it is not unreasonable to assume the problem is part of a general social attitude. Where the pattern is long-standing, but not common to the family of origin, it is worth considering the possibility of mental illness or of severe emotional disturbance. Where the pattern is long-standing but was preceded by a good work record, it is vital to try and understand what caused the deterioration. The reason may have been abrupt and traumatic. It is not uncommon, for example, for the difficulty to stem from redundancy which gave the man a severe blow to his morale. The man's age at such a time is frequently crucial to his success in finding alternative employment and will in any case affect his adjustment to the situation. Or, again common in case records, the deterioration may have begun at the time of marriage and be related to increased demands of the family or marital difficulties. Another work pattern that may present even more difficulties to social workers and officials than the long-standing unemployed is that of men who are always 'off and on' the books, with short spells of employment. We do not know enough about this. (It is one of the problems being examined in the current research project.) It will be interesting to know more of the details of such 'job behaviour', for example, if on occasions there is a recurrent pattern, such as quarrelling with the foreman. Such information might have practical treatment implications. The findings of Martin and Webster are relevant to this problem.[1] In their study groups, 'criminals' and bad

[1] J. P. Martin and P. Webster. *Social Consequences of Conviction*, Heinemann, London, 1971.

drivers were compared. Job instability was very high among the former in comparison with the latter. Particular reference was made to the question of self employment. 'Self employment . . . is related to what seems to be an important characteristic of some offenders. This was a strong dislike of having to work for others and to obey instructions.' The study revealed that the criminals were not more likely than the bad drivers to have tried working on their own but that they were far more likely to have tried more than twice. The study suggests that the criminals may have been less successful than the bad drivers in their attempts to work on their own.

Work Stresses

No study of voluntary unemployment would be complete if it focused solely on the individual and his relations with his family, past and present, and left out of account the stresses to which a working man is exposed, which vary in different types of employment. It may be that there is something intrinsically harsh and frightening in the work itself with which a number of men simply cannot cope. The coal-mining industry is an obvious example and the problem has been recognised by some experienced officers in mining areas. (In a survey of men prosecuted, 14 per cent were, or had been, miners.) Much more needs to be known in cases of so-called 'voluntary unemployment' about the men's reactions to the particular work available. Difficulties also arise, however, in working relationships. Not only relationships with authority are important but also the man's relationships with peers. It would not be surprising to learn that some of the inadequate and unattractive men, who comprise a number of the voluntarily unemployed, have opted out of situations where they have been constantly mocked and 'had the mickey taken'. Yet these are the kinds of experiences rarely revealed, perhaps because they are too humiliating, perhaps because of the fear that they will be rejected as excuses. Consider, for example, a car assembly line, in which men work in groups at piece-work rates. This necessitates a close working relationship with a small number of men and upon this the level of earnings depends. A weak link will therefore be much resented. Furthermore, the work-flow is uneven—there are periods of inactivity followed by intense bursts of activity at uneven intervals. This may be better tolerated by some individuals than others but is inclined to generate tension in all concerned. Analysis of these and other work situations would reveal the kinds of difficulty inherent in the work itself or in the relationships connected with it, which some men cannot tolerate.

Discussion of this kind is not intended to minimise the practical difficulties that may exist for supplementary benefits claimants even in areas of high employment. Men with criminal records may have particular difficulties in certain areas. For example, in Plymouth most of the available work is in H.M. dockyards which will not accept such men. However, it is worth noting in this connection the comments of Martin and Webster[1] concerning their 'criminal' group:

'The apparent infrequency of sacking men for the discovery of their criminal careers is less surprising. The general level of unemployment was low, tending to be unskilled or casual and the rate of change of jobs was high in any event. While we have no doubt that there are circumstances under which men lose their jobs because of their records, they are probably not very common at the level on which most of the men worked on release.'

Yet even without a criminal record a man may become well known, if not notorious, in a particular area. This can lead to a situation where, partly through the realities of past experience and partly through moral outrage and 'a scape-goating' process, the man becomes a social pariah and would probably be unemployable even if he had a change of heart. This is particularly likely to happen in areas where employment is not diversified. There is a vicious circle in this which has been observed in work with problem families generally. The problems create hostility in local society. This in turn creates more problems and reinforces the feeling of the family that 'all the world is against them'. Even without this direct social ostracism, however, which is more likely to be felt in the rural or more closeknit urban areas, it has to be acknowledged that such claimants are going to be at the bottom of an employer's list and may only be taken on in areas of exceptionally *high* employment.

The aim of this discussion has been to suggest the complexity of the factors involved. It is hoped that the research now in progress may give some idea as to whether the analysis is reasonably accurate and comprehensive, and of the relative importance of different factors involved. The following illustration serves to remind us that behind the theoretical frames of reference and the statistics are the people, whose circumstances may be both complicated and pitiful.

'Mr B is now 30 years old. He has three children. Attempts have been made to get him to attend an Industrial Rehabilitation Unit, but he

[1] Op. cit.

returned home "because of his wife's emotional state". His wife has disseminated sclerosis and is largely confined to a wheel-chair. A doctor found him to have no present disability . . . nothing physical or psychological to necessitate registration as a disabled person. He was fit for his own job as a welder. In the face of continued unemployment, he was seen by a psychiatrist who reported: "At interview, the patient said that he did not feel that there was any basic reason why, mentally or physically, he should be unable to work." However, he made the following points:

He said he can only take labouring jobs but is often turned down because he is so small. This is quite correct—he is very short and weighs under eight stone. He had, he said, never been properly trained and could not cope with automation which the firm introduced a few years ago. In this connection, it is interesting to note that he was in stable employment for more than five years until automation was introduced. However, the poor work record also coincides with the time of his marriage: he has taken time off to keep his wife and lost his job. He says his wife is very nervous about being left in the house alone and that relatives and friends vary in the amount they are willing to help her. She had quarrelled with her mother who used to spend much time in the house.'

CHAPTER 5

VOLUNTARY UNEMPLOYMENT II— INVESTIGATION AND TREATMENT

'All public income security systems dealing with presumably employable persons pay great attention to tests of the involuntary character of claimants alleged inability to earn.' (Burns, 1956)[1]

'I was called up there before that fellow to answer for my sins whatever they were. I guess I had been out of work too long. As if it was my fault. But anyway, there I stood. "Sit down", he says, just like that he says to me, "Sit down". So I sat down on the chair there in front of him. He went on writing, and me wondering what he was going to say. Then he looked at me sort of lazy-like and says, "Where were you yesterday?" That was Tuesday. I told him several places. Then he says, "Where were you looking for work Monday?" I told him some more. "Where were you Sunday?" He knew he had no business asking that one, but I answered right back, "I read the newspapers to see if I could find where any help was needed." Not everyone would have thought of that, mate. But I have always been quick like that, I had to be. Then he said, "Where were you Saturday?" I gave him the names of some other places. "Where were you Friday?" By that time I had some trouble in thinking where I had been, but I managed to tell him a couple more. Then quick-like he looked straight at me and says, "Where were you yesterday?" I saw he was trying to trick me, so I says, "I just told you that and if you took it down you've got it." He told me not to get saucy. And I told him that I didn't like him trying to trip me up that way. He said that he guessed I didn't show I was honestly wanting to work and sent me out. I expected to have my benefit stopped, but it wasn't. How do you account for that?'

This account by Bakke[2] described an encounter with a Labour Exchange official in the thirties. Bakke continues:

---

[1] E. Burns, *The American Social Security System,* Houghton Miffler, New York, 1951.
[2] Bakke, op. cit.

'Possibly one may "account for that" by merely saying that the officer was not trying to trick him at all, but was taking the easiest way of "making conversation" without any malevolent intent: but the interviewed man sees this questioning in the light of his fears and of assumptions deriving, I suspect, from popular belief as to the nature and practice of interviewing before the abolition of the "genuinely seeking work" classes. Interviewing so conducted, at the time to which this record relates, would have been entirely contrary to instructions. But in matters of social administration, beliefs about facts are themselves facts to reckon with; and since the initial determination of eligibility for benefit rests upon the impression formed by the interviewing officer, these beliefs count for much in the minds and attitudes of the unemployed.'

Policies and procedures have changed since then but the essentials remain. The administration continues to seek to persuade men to work, and, as Bakke points out 'beliefs about facts are themselves facts to reckon with'. The rest of this chapter will be mainly concerned with the ways in which the Supplementary Benefits Commission exercises its responsibilities. The difficulties it has in doing so have already been implied by the preceding chapter. Two preliminary issues need to be explored further; first, the implication of the 'requirement to register for work' and, second, the role of the Department of Employment and Productivity in relation to these men.

Registration for Employment

Whatever concern there may be about 'the voluntarily unemployed' as a social problem for the official the core of the difficulty is administrative. That is to say, whatever his private views may be about a particular claimant he is absolved from any responsibility to encourage the man to work if the statutory requirement to register for work is waived.

'The Commission have power to decide that payment of supplementary allowances shall be subject to the condition that a person register for work ... This rule is normally applied to anyone who is capable of work but it does not apply to a claimant for supplementary pension—that is to say, a man over 65 or a woman over 60.
    Claimants who are not required to register include:

1. People who are incapable of work—based on medical evidence of incapacity.

2. Women who have dependent children under 16 living with them.
3. Blind persons who have not been accustomed to working outside the home.

For certain other groups of people the requirement to register may be waived or registration for part-time work only may be required. Depending on the circumstances of the case these include:

1. People required at home to care for sick relatives.
2. Women widowed in later middle life with no experience in the employment field and where there is some evidence of ill-health.
3. People on (certain) training or other educational courses.'[1]

At the time of writing, further instructions concerning registration have just been issued and these are not included in the Handbook.[2] Briefly, these make it possible for certain claimants to sign on quarter-yearly at the Employment Exchange. This measure, while not, of course, waiving the requirement, makes the duty much less onerous than the former 'weekly trip' and has many advantages. It was some-times argued by officials that some claiments whose chances of employ-ment were slim preferred to continue to register weekly since it gave them hope—albeit a false one—of a normal life. This is open to doubt, however. The new 'quarterly signing' procedures leave claimants with some hope of employment but, both administratively and psychologically, should be more satisfactory. It should be noted, however, that no-one required to register, at *whatever intervals*, qualifies for the 'long term addition'.[3]

The latest instructions permit quarterly signing for men of 55 years of age or over 50 for women who have been unemployed for at least two years, provided that during the last two years there had been no instance of fraud or 'voluntary unemployment'. These cases are identified by the Employment Exchange and referred to local Supplementary Benefits offices for consideration; no judgement is called for concerning the likelihood of an early placing in employment. Quarterly signing is also considered for those whose prospects of employment are handicapped due to physical disability, mental disability or age, and who have been unemployed for at least one year. Similar conditions about fraud and voluntary unemployment also apply but a judgement is required in each individual case as to the likelihood of an early placing in employment. These cases are identi-

[1] See Supplementary Benefits Handbook, Paras 6–8.
[2] The Handbook is regularly revised. A 3rd edition is pending.
[3] The LTA is at present 50p per week.

fied by local Supplementary Benefits offices who seek advice from
Employment Exchanges.

While there is no doubt that the intention of these provisions is
humane, as well as administratively sensible, they highlight some of
the problems of discretionary power discussed earlier.[1] It is clear, for
example, that decisions, whether by the Employment Exchange or the
SB local office, about quarterly registration, will depend upon past
judgements about voluntary unemployment and on present judgements about the extent of mental and physical handicap. It is too early
yet to say how effective the instructions will be in practice.

Whatever the arguments for continued registering, some men whose
chances of employment are extremely slim may find themselves in an
ambiguous position. Officers may have grave doubts as to whether
they can work but repetitive advice is often given that they should do
so, sometimes no doubt with helpful interest, sometimes to satisfy
what is felt to be an obligation. It cannot be said with certainty that
this is damaging to claimants; they may get so inured to it that they
scarcely hear. Yet there is something distasteful about a situation in
which officers feel obliged to encourage claimants to get a job when
they doubt if in fact there is a job he could get.

Even more unfortunate, however, is the situation of men who,
according to the present system, are not considered to be suffering
from a mental or physical handicap sufficient to waive the requirement
to register altogether but who are already inadequate in many ways or
whose family circumstances present insuperable difficulties to their
taking work. The difficulty is that until more sophisticated methods of
help have been tried and systematically evaluated we cannot say with
certainty how many are totally unemployable. In any case, as war-
time conditions of full employment showed, this is dependent to a
considerable extent on the demand for labour. Furthermore, 'unem-
ployability' will be related to technological changes that reduce the
need for unskilled labour. It would be rash, therefore, to suggest
greater flexibility in the registration requirements unless, and until,
there is a corresponding development in investigation and treatment,
and without taking into account fluctuations and fundamental changes
in the labour market. It would be deplorable if a number of men were,
in effect, put on the scrap heap who might, given suitable support, be
maintained in employment. The development of increased facilities
for sheltered and protected employment may be an essential consequence of technological advance. Furthermore, a practical difficulty

[1] See Chapter 2.

of considerable importance arises in that if a man is *neither* registered for employment *nor* certified as sick, he is not entitled to National Insurance Credits. This is true at present for men who are not always required to register when they stay at home to look after children. (The National Insurance regulations for woman are, of course, different.)

Apropos of family circumstances, it is interesting and regrettable to note that although the Supplementary Benefits Handbook refers to the possibility of waiving registration for '*people*', i.e. of either sex 're-quired at home to care for sick relatives or *women* (my italics) who have dependent children under 16 living with them',[1] it does not refer at that stage to the possibility of men caring for dependent children. However, a later paragraph makes it clear that, at least in the initial stages, requirement to register can be waived in such cases: 'If the father himself gives up work to care for his sick wife or for his young children during the illness or unavoidable absence of their mother, the Commission will normally pay him a supplementary allowance without requiring him to register for work, to tide him over the immediate emergency, provided it is clear that no satisfactory alterna-tive is available'.[2] The Handbook goes on to discuss what should be done in the long term but it is not clear how usual it would be to insist on registration after the emergency period (although officers are instructed to take the views of social workers seriously into account). Further, although the earlier paragraph speaks of *people* looking after sick relatives, a later paragraph speaks only of *women* in general terms as not being required to register in such circumstances. For men the provisions are much more restricted and more ambiguous in their application.[3] It is hard to avoid the conclusion that the provisions as a whole discriminate against men and may involve officials and claimants in awkward situations in which the requirement to register is depen-dent on assessment of highly complex situations involving value judgements. This double standard for men and women accords oddly with contemporary trends in which men take an increasing share in domestic activities. It may be argued that it should be just as accep-table socially for a man to care for his sick wife as for a woman to care for her mother and that no formal distinction in terms of registration for work should be made. As against this, the Commission's view is that it will usually be in the best interest of the family as a whole for a man to get back to work, although it is recognised that there will be exceptions. In these two not uncommon situations of men caring for

[1] Supplementary Benefits Handbook, para. 8 (1).   [2] Ibid., para. 134 (2).
[3] Ibid., paras. 132 and 134.

children or sick wives we see an interesting and controversial example
of the ways in which policy mirrors, or seeks to mirror, the social
values of the time and the difficulties for those who frame policy in
assessing these.

Any further revision of the existing practice would need the combined expertise of professionals such as doctors and social workers and
administrators and would undoubtedly be complex and time-consuming. As a starting-point to the consideration of the treatment of
unemployed men, however, it is vital. The wide discretionary powers
at present available to Supplementary Benefits officials might be
constructively limited if 'requirement to register' were more frequently
waived. In particular it would be useful to attempt to construct a
formula in which social and family circumstances or more subtle forms
of personal difficulty or inadequacy would be taken into accord in the
waiving of registration requirements.

Relations with the Department of Employment and Productivity

This raises the question of aspects of the relationship of the SBC to the
DEP. As the scheme stands, men receive a supplementary allowance
when they are not eligible for unemployment benefit—for example
when they have been dismissed for misconduct, when their title to
unemployment benefit is exhausted or when they have insufficient
stamps. (They may, of course, also receive an allowance as a supplement to unemployment benefit.) Thus it is inevitable that among the
unemployed men claiming a supplementary allowance there will be a
higher proportion of 'difficult cases' than among those only claiming
unemployment benefit. This division of responsibility, however, is
not without its complications. First, if it is true as is frequently
suggested, that attempts to help unemployed men are more likely
to succeed earlier than later, those men who, at the beginning of
their period of unemployment, receive unemployment benefit and
whose contact is therefore with DEP officials will be affected by the
treatment they receive there in the early stages. Subsequent intervention by Supplementary Benefits officials may be more or less
effective because of this. Secondly, it has become apparent that, of
recent years, the DEP has been less interested in the men who fall into
this category than in those whose unemployment is solely due to
market forces and who have good prospects of resettlement. This is
understandable in the light of the concern of the DEP to improve their
image with employers and employees and to avoid a situation in
which employers frequently bypass the Department in recruiting

labour. Many of the men with whom these chapters have been concerned are unattractive employment propositions and the DEP risks jeopardising its relations with employers by presenting them. This to some extent explains the fact that the SBC has itself devised measures to deal with the problem. Despite the fact that, at first glance, it seems illogical, even wasteful, for the Commission to extend and develop its functions in this sphere, there seems to be little alternative unless, as will be discussed later, the social work services were to become more closely involved. The reality seems to be that the SBC is more likely to concern itself with this small but time-consuming group of men than the DEP.

SBC Policy and Practice

We move now to consider the policy and practice of the SBC in relation to its work with unemployed men, focusing mainly upon those whose presenting symptoms suggest to the officials that their unemployment might be due to their own choice.

It is clear from the examination of instructions to officials and the ways in which training has developed over the past years that official policy towards those who are on the margins of employability has become progressively more humane, despite certain aspects of it, such as 'the four week rule', which have attracted criticism in some quarters. This is shown by a greater and more detailed emphasis on the problem such individuals have in getting and obtaining work, and the many exceptions and qualifications to the rules concerning restriction or refusal of benefit to unemployed men. It is important in this, as in so many other aspects of Supplementary Benefits administration (as indeed in other spheres of public administration), to distinguish clearly between declared policy and the actuality of practice. But if a wide gap is seen to exist between the two, it is simplistic to explain the gap by suggesting that declared policy is insincere and designed 'to whitewash the facts'. Developments and changes in policy take a considerable time to be effectively implemented, bearing in mind the problems of manpower, staff training, and above all, the nature of bureaucratic organisations.[1] What may be questionable, however, is the assumption that the very detailed instructions needed to protect claimants and the relatively sophisticated approaches to claimants needed to implement some of them *can* be effectively carried through by officials employed within the constraints of the present Supplementary Benefits organisation and staff resources. To understand this

[1] See Chapter 3.

better, we must examine in some detail Supplementary Benefits policy with regard to unemployed men generally.

Over and over again in official documents the importance of observing and making allowances for physical and/or mental handicaps is stressed. The safeguards to the claimant (rights of appeal, referral to higher authority, etc.) are also emphasised. The 'standard control' procedures laid down by the SBC fall into two categories; those that are routine—that is to say, those that apply to all unemployed claimants; and those that are only applicable when voluntary unemployment is suspected.

Control Procedures

The first consists of ordinary review visits to older unemployed claimants in receipt of a supplementary allowance, the frequency of these being determined by the age of the men and women; and certain special restrictions of the duration of the allowance for younger claimants. One of these is the widely publicised 'four week rule'.

The Four Week Rule

This applies to certain unskilled claimants between the ages of 18 and 45 who live in areas in which it has been agreed with the DEP that they have good job opportunities. Under this rule benefit may be given for four weeks only at the outset of the claim. If the claim is renewed at the end of that period, it may be discontinued (if circumstances are unaltered) subject, of course, to the right of appeal. However the rule is subject to many qualifications, the details of which cannot be enumerated here. For example, pregnant women and claimants with serious physical or mental disability are excluded. Also excluded are those who are described as 'socially inadequate' in ways likely to lessen their chances of employment. This term, however imprecise, increases considerably the range of claimants to whom the rule may not be applied. Claimants with dependent children are also excluded and the need for careful consideration of the likelihood of a *particular* claimant being offered work is urged (for example, a man with a serious prison record). The rule is intended to apply only to unskilled labourers since it is acknowledged that skilled or semi-skilled men may take longer to find suitable work.

The number of men at present involved in this procedure is relatively small; at the time of writing only 3·6 per cent of the running orders issued at the Employment Exchange are subject to a four week limitation, and the percentage of these in which a decision is taken to terminate benefit is smaller still. Perhaps the careful instructions play a part in keeping these numbers small. They certainly imply a recognition by the Commission of the risks of inappropriate limitation of benefit. Even so it seems inevitable that certain individuals will suffer to a considerable extent if the local administration has not the time, the skill or the inclination to probe such matters at the early stages of a claim.

Three Month Reviews

A second stage in the standard control procedure is the review after three months. This applies to other claimants under 45 and includes skilled workers. In such cases, subject to many of the same safeguards as have been outlined above and some additional ones, a renewed allowance may at that stage be limited to four weeks.

These procedures, then, are intended to be of general application at two stages during unemployment. They are relevant to the problem under consideration because they give an indication of the ways in which policies, if effectively carried through, would contribute, on the one hand, to reasonable control of abuse and, on the other, to the avoidance of undue pressure on some men and to greater understanding of the factors that are responsible for or are likely to contribute to their difficulties in obtaining work.

Control of Voluntary Unemployment

Within the more restricted definition of the term as used by officials 'voluntary unemployment' is indicated if a person has left a job within the preceding six weeks without good cause, because of industrial misconduct, or if he has refused an offer of suitable employment without good reason. One notes the large element of subjectivity in the perception by employers and employees, Employment Exchange and Supplementary Benefits officials which makes such assumptions fraught with difficulty. For example, it is particularly difficult to disentangle the rights and wrongs of situations in which men have provoked their own dismissal or been provoked by others to encourage them to leave.

Once 'voluntary unemployment' in a particular case is suspected, there are four main forms of control. These are the restriction or withdrawal of benefit; intervention by an Unemployment Review Officer; attendance at a Re-establishment Centre; and prosecution.

However, although these are described as procedures of control, the second and third in particular may also contain positive factors designed to help the men involved.

Restriction or Withdrawal of Benefit

Reduced allowances may be paid or, exceptionally, refused. However, as with the controls discussed previously, this discretionary power is hedged round with qualifications. Supplementary Benefit may be temporarily restricted pending a decision by the Insurance Officer concerning eligibility to unemployment benefit. In such cases, guidance is given to officials in the interpretation of the phrases 'without good cause' or 'without good reason' used in connection with giving up work. For example they are reminded that dismissal for absence may be explicable in terms of domestic difficulties or of the claimant's anxiety in a particular job (such as fear of heights). Similarly, refusal of work may be explicable in particular circumstances, as when there are considerable transport difficulties in getting to the job. Instructions are even more cautious if more stringent consideration is given to the refusal or withdrawal of a supplementary allowance, when unemployment benefit is disallowed. Thus a suitable job must be immediately available or there must have been previous incidents of voluntary unemployment and there must be ample work in the area; and the physical, mental, and family circumstances of the claimant must be taken into account. All this affords a particularly vivid illustration both of the inevitability of, but also the limits upon, the exercise of discretion. The detailed guidance which is given seeks to control the extent of the variations between officials. Helpful and humane as it is, however, it cannot, and could not ever, remove the need for careful and unbiased judgement on the part of the official. In any case it is an attempt to formulate with greater precision policies that deal in large measure with imprecise, complex, subtle and subjective processes of human interaction, at work and at home. This is the nub of the administrative dilemma.

Intervention by Unemployment Review Officers

The role and function of the UROs have been described briefly in an earlier chapter and it has been suggested that there may be conflicts for them in carrying these out. Recent instructions to UROS, as in other aspects of 'voluntary unemployment', have laid increasing emphasis on the importance of seeking to understand and help such men, which may lessen some aspects of this role conflict. The conflicts that may now be sharpest, however, may be between Headquarters policy and local office attitudes, or in some cases, those in the URO himself. Certainly there is nothing in instructions to discourage UROs from taking an active and informed interest in the problems of his claimants; on the contrary, the spirit as well as the detail of Headquarters policy can hardly be faulted, if one accepts the premise on which they are based, i.e. that 'voluntary unemployment' exists and that administrative efforts must be made to control it.

As indicated earlier, the numbers of UROs have been expanded and the following approximate figures give some indication of the extent of their activity in the six months up to June 1971. In the country as a whole (including Scotland) 24,200 claimants were called for interview by regionally-based UROs. Of these, 18,500 were in fact interviewed while some 4,500 (19 per cent) went off the books before the interview. There were 34,500 interviews. This averages out at scarcely more than two interviews per claimant, although a smaller number of claimants may, of course, have been seen very frequently, particularly as we know that 5,600 (23 per cent) obtained work after one interview. Another 1,400 (6 per cent) had the allowance withdrawn with or without direct contact with the URO.

There are also figures available for officials in local offices performing the role of URO. In the same period 41,300 were called for interview; 34,100 claimants were interviewed, while 6,500 (16 per cent) went off the books before interview. There were 47,200 interviews—proportionally a much smaller number than in the case of regionally-based UROs. However, a much higher proportion, 14,500 (34 per cent), are said to have obtained work after one interview and slightly more, 3,300 (8 per cent), had their allowance withdrawn with or without direct contact with officials.

These figures as a whole reveal some interesting aspects of the problem. For example, it will not surprise the Supplementary Benefits administrator that between 15 per cent and 20 per cent of claimants called for interview did not attend and went off the books. It must be a matter for concern that amongst these there will be a number who have ceased to claim but are not in fact self-supporting. They may, for example, be living on the allowances paid to relatives or living below subsistence level. It is certain, however, that there will also be those who have decided to take work or who have had undeclared sources of additional income all along, 'earning on the side'. There is no evidence what the proportions are of each. Common sense suggests that in some areas, especially those in which casual employment is easy to come by, there will be quite a substantial proportion of the latter. But social workers are properly concerned, whatever the numbers involved, if the former are deterred from claiming their entitlement through fear of an interview in prospect. The figures also indicate that the unemployed man does not usually have frequent or prolonged contact with the URO. Many will not need or want such contact but it is important that social workers should appreciate the limited nature of this intervention at the present time.

The UROs or their specially designed equivalents in local offices have a threefold task, according to instructions. First, they should assess the climant's capacity for work as an individual *and* in relation to work available in the area. Secondly, they should attempt to diagnose why the claimant is not working through interview, records, consultation with others and so on. In this they should take into account the factors that have been outlined in the previous chapter. Thirdly, they should seek for ways of solving the problem or improving the situation. They should not interview claimants for whom employment seems a remote possibility or impossible (for example, older people, those registered as disabled, and so on).

At the stage of assessment interviews, UROs are required to inquire into the claimant's situation in considerable depth and what is now expected of them is not dissimilar to the task of the Probation Officer in making a social inquiry report. (They are also encouraged to give men a good deal of help and to refer them to social workers whenever desirable.) This raises the question of the competence of officials to undertake their task. Assessment interviews of this kind are unlikely to be highly successful if they are in the form of structured questionnaires; but open-ended interviews require a basic understanding of the justification for, and meaning of, the questions. Furthermore, such detailed questions are very different from the unemployed man's normal contact with the Supplementary Benefits official and the claimant's expectations are bound to affect the situation. Until 1970, the UROs received no special training and were specialist only in terms of role and not as a result of any particular expertise, except that acquired from experience on the job. The recognition of the need for some specialist training was a milestone in the development of the policy towards the voluntarily unemployed. Its superficiality, in terms of length (two weeks) compared with that of social workers, is obvious. But this should not be allowed to overshadow the fundamental significance of the innovation that implies an acceptance that the task cannot be effectively performed without certain knowledge going beyond that which the official can expect to possess 'by the light of nature'. The development of such training is consistent with the attitudes of the old National Assistance Board to the problem. Conscious of their dilemma, the National Assistance Board gave more attention to this problem in basic training of executive and clerical officers than to any other. The present specialist courses run by a Department of Social Work at a university met with some initial (and almost traditional) scepticism by the UROs; but subsequently they made full use of the courses, revealing anxiety and concern about their claimants and their own role and a keen desire to learn more of the factors associated with voluntary unemployment. This enlightened policy on the part of the SBC may, however, boomerang. For such courses are bound to raise questions in the minds of officials about the way in which their role has been defined and the opportunity—or lack of opportunity—it offers to exercise certain skills, akin to social work, about which they learn in training.

Recent trends, therefore, in the SBC have tended to move the UROs along a road towards social work. This, in the writer's opinion, is desirable in that it indicates not only an increased sympathy for the unemployed man but also an increased willingness to study those factors underlying the problems which must be understood if the sympathy is to be informed. Such a movement, however, is not without its problems for two reasons: first, as had been indicated, role conflicts for some officials might become intolerable if expectations were raised which they could not fulfil because of the way in which their work is organised and the limitations of their training. Secondly, the efficacy of social work intervention in general[1] and in relation to unemployed men in particular is as yet unproven. The objective of the action research now under way is to compare the effectiveness of different groups in re-establishing men in employment.[2] The three groups to be studied are: the UROs as at present trained and deployed; 'special' UROs who are given more social work advice; and qualified social workers. The outcome may have significant implications for policy. One thing is certain; as has been demonstrated by the discussion in the preceding chapter, the assessment and help offered to the unemployed man cannot need *less* skill than that needed by social workers in dealing with comparable problems. That is not to say they all need it: it is simply to emphasise that, as with social work with

[1] See, for example, M. Goldberg, *Helping the Aged*, Allen & Unwin, London, 1971.
[2] See Appendix II.

other groups, to know when and when not such skill is required in individual cases is in itself a skill.

Re-establishment Centres

'The Commission . . . run centres "for the re-establishment of persons in need thereof through lack of regular occupation or of instruction or training" in order to fit them for entry into or return to regular employment. There are thirteen such centres; three have residential facilities; and they all have facilities for men in the surrounding areas to attend daily.[1]

In the period 1966–1970 an average of 1,700 men attended Re-establishment Centres each year. In general social workers have little knowledge of the existence of these facilities and still less of the way they operate. Furthermore, Re-establishment Centres function in a considerable degree of isolation from other forms of 'day and residential care', with which they have much in common. Thus they afford a useful illustration of the problems arising from the separation of income maintenance services from the 'personal' social services.

Most Re-establishment Centres are housed alongside the Reception Centres provided for men 'without a settled way of living'. There are certain advantages to this arrangement, the main one being that employment facilities are open to both. Thus the advantage is mainly to the Reception Centre which at times offers shelter for a period of months and can use the Re-establishment Centre to further its statutory duty 'to make provision whereby persons without a settled way of living may be influenced to lead a more settled life'.[2] The advantage to the Re-establishment Centre is less clear, except insofar as their co-existence makes possible the appointment of an officer of higher grade as Manager. It may be that there are disadvantages if men who come, or are asked to come, feel to some extent stigmatised by association with the clientele of the Reception Centres. We have no evidence on this point but officials suggest that there is considerable mutual antagonism.

The vast majority of men who attend Re-establishment Centres do so voluntarily, although there are powers to direct them to do so.[3] The absence of statutory constraint does not mean, of course, that every man who attends a Re-establishment Centre goes willingly. He may

[1] See Supplementary Benefits Handbook, Para. 179.
[2] Social Security Act, 1966, Section 34.
[3] Ministry of Social Security Act, 1966, Section II.

go as a result of strong pressure or encouragement from the local office and, on occasions, may fear—reasonably or unreasonably—that if he does not and remains unemployed, some action, such as prosecution, will be taken against him. At other times, however, especially in areas in which employment is difficult, men are said to want to go, believing that it may increase their chances of getting a job. For those who are 'involuntary volunteers' the familiar issues of social control, discussed earlier in this book, are raised. In principle, the 'involuntary volunteer' at the Re-establishment Centre is no different from the probationer who accepts the order as an alternative to something worse. It would be hypocritical for social workers to criticise the Re-establishment Centres on these grounds. But as in all forms of treatment, this fact does have a bearing on the workings of the Re-establishment Centre, affecting as it does the motivation of the men who attend them. As in social work it places the onus on the staff of the Centre to provide facilities and establish relationships so that the motivation of the man to attend and to gain employment is increased even in the face of initial reluctance.

The declared aim of the Re-establishment Centres is to provide routine employment of an unskilled or semi-skilled variety to encourage men to get back into the habit of regular work. The Department of Employment and Productivity has been defined as responsible for job training; hence the choice of the phrase 'Re-establishment Centre' in contrast, for example, to that of 'Industrial Rehabilitation Unit'. At present most of the work provided within the Re-establishment Centres is relatively unsophisticated—woodwork paying a large part— and any substantial change towards more elaborate industrial activities would require not only considerable capital expenditure and more technically skilled staff but also an acceptance by the Commission of a role in matters of employment, which has been thought of as belonging to the DEP. It is clear that at present Re-establishment Centres take men who would not be accepted for any specialised DEP provision and who have, by any standards, marginal employment prospects. Managers often make great efforts to find the men a job at the end of their stay; and their support also includes discussion of family problems and other associated difficulties. The Manager of a combined Re-establishment and Reception Centre is usually a Higher Executive Officer; that is to say, this is his first promotion above Executive Officer. He is likely to have applied and to have been selected for this post because of a particular interest in the problem. Until recently no special training was provided for the work but since 1971 short courses of two weeks are being arranged for all Managers of Reception Centres and their staff.[1] The writer visited a number of Re-establishment Centres and formed the impression that much constructive and compassionate effort was being made by individual officers to help the men at their Centres. Nevertheless, however well-intentioned the efforts of many involved in the work of the Centres, their very existence raises some important questions and problems for the SBC.

First, there is the question of evaluating their success. There seems little doubt that, in view of the extremely poor work records of many men who are admitted, the Re-establishment Centres achieve a creditable number of successes, measured in terms of men obtaining employment on discharge, particularly as the Re-establishment Centre is mostly used as a last resort. (The figures indicate that between 40 and 50 per cent do so.) What is not clear is whether a number of those men could be helped equally well outside the Centres if skilled and sustained support in the community were available; such support is rarely available. In other words, the significant element in success achieved thus far has not been identified. Does it lie in the regular routine of the Centre, training in regular work, mixing with peers, and having to leave home each morning? Or does it lie in the relationships created and the efforts made by Managers to find men employment which include relationships made by them with employers? It is, of course, extremely important to know this because of the implications for future developments. Is the expensive paraphenalia of a Re-establishment Centre necessary? It may be so but we do not know. Furthermore, evaluation of success must, of course, be refined or extended. At the very least there should be information as to how many men who gain employment on discharge lose it again within a stated period.

Secondly, the Re-establishment Centres have to be examined within the context of developments in the social services as a whole. They have a constructive and, on the whole, benign approach to their task. Yet, until recently, the assumption has been made that the task is one for which ordinary administrative skills are sufficient, together with the common sense and humanity of the 'ordinary man'. Further, it should be noted, the running of a combined Reception and Re-establishment Centre is entrusted to an officer of comparatively low rank. (A Re-establishment Centre on its own would only qualify for an Executive Officer as Manager). This is not to say that there are not excellent and devoted officers in post. But it gives an indication of the

[1] See Chapter 8.

value the organisation places upon the skills needed. Social workers, drawing parallels with, for example, wardens of probation hostels or the superintendent of a day centre for the mentally ill, will readily appreciate the kinds of skill and training that are likely to be relevant to the work of the Re-establishment Centres and the manifold opportunities for experiment they offer. It is doubtful whether such experiments could ever develop as freely within the present structure as one might wish. It is in the nature of a strongly bureaucratic structure that the impetus for experiment and change in such matters is often lacking. For the Re-establishment Centres are not in the mainstream of rehabilitative work although their functions would justify their being so. Their staff have had little contact with others in related work and, inevitably, there is no sense of common identity arising from an identified professional skill. These difficulties are likely to become more significant in the next few years for two reasons. One is that the limited training now being offered to the staff of the re-establishment centres will begin to widen horizons and create more anxiety about what they do not know. (This is, of course, no reason for not offering it.) The second is that the social services as a whole are becoming aware of the skills involved in forms of residential and day care and the need for extended provisions of this kind. Hopefully these will develop fast. This could increase the gap between professionally and administratively orientated provision, although the SBC's increased openness to professional expertise may avert this. In fact a strong case could be made for the appointment of social workers to run these Centres especially, of course, since so many are combined with Reception Centres. The earlier view of the social worker as a person skilled in casework and not necessarily in the management of therapeutically orientated establishments dies hard and it is understandable that the SBC is as yet uncertain as to the role they might play. Indeed, social work as a whole has only recently begun to widen its own definition of professional function.

Thirdly, the relationship of the Re-establishment Centres to their own local offices needs consideration. At present, the work of the Re-establishment Centres is not effectively integrated with that of the local office. There is an understandable tendency for the local office staff, temporarily relieved of the responsibility for a claimant who has probably been a source of considerable anxiety or annoyance, to opt out. (Social workers will not be unfamiliar with this in their own work.) Equally or more important, however, is that the organisation does not expect or assume that there will be continuity of concern as might a good social service department. Thus, it may happen that a man who, on discharge from the Re-establishment Centre, gets work but needs support in keeping it, or who fails to get work, will not receive help of the kind he may have received at the Centre once he is back in the community. Furthermore, it was the impression of the writer that the relevant 'specialists' within the SBC—the Special Welfare Officers and the Unemployment Review Officers—had surprisingly little to do with the Re-establishment Centres. In short, the Re-establishment Centres suffer, as do a number of significant 'welfare elements' within the SBC, from a considerable degree of internal structural isolation, as a result of lack of *continuity of planning*, in this case for the treatment of the unemployed man.

Lastly there is the matter of contact with social workers at field level. In this one must distinguish between the claimants who attend the Re-establishment Centre daily from their homes (or who are specifically referred to the two residential Re-establishment Centres) and those who work in the Re-establishment Centre and are living in the adjacent Reception Centre. As far as the former are concerned it seems reasonable to assume that in many cases liasion between the SBC and the social service departments or other agencies will be highly desirable, since it is likely that there will be a number of associated problems and that the claimant has an intact family to which he returns. At present Re-establishment Centres make little direct contact with social workers, the channel of communication being via the local office. It seems desirable that the staff of the Centre should feel free to make direct contact in cases in which there are immediate family and social problems relevant to the problem of unemployment.

Many of the men in the Reception Centres are, of course, rootless and transient and in such cases effective liasion is much more difficult to achieve. The many thorny issues raised by Reception Centres are, regrettably, outside the scope of this book. In general, however, the writer observed that the work of Re-establishment Centres was virtually unknown to social workers. It seems extremely important that social workers should be better informed, both generally and in relation to particular local centres, about this aspect of the Commission's responsibilities.

There seems little doubt that the Re-establishment Centres have a contribution to make to the study and treatment of the long-term unemployed. However before we can be sure of the nature of that contribution much more needs to be known about them, not only in evaluative terms but also in terms of the processes within the centres:

for example, how men are assessed on admission; the time spent and methods employed in interviewing; the nature of the contacts with employers. In the longer term it seems vital that Re-establishment Centres should find their way into the mainstream of residential and day care for adults who have social problems. Whether this can be done if they remain within the orbit of the SBC (for example, by the appointment of social workers to run them or by increased use of professional expertise) or whether they need to be taken into social service agencies who will have a growing experience of a range of similar provisions remains to be seen. It should be emphasised, however, that the learning is not one-way, between social workers and the SBC. Much useful experience has been gained by the Re-establishment Centre staff in the rehabilitation of unemployed men from which social workers can profit.

Prosecution

The Supplementary Benefits Commission have powers to prosecute men who, it is alleged, have refused or neglected to maintain themselves and their dependents. Prosecution is sparingly used and decisions to initiate it are always taken at Headquarters. The decision is taken following a number of incidents of refusal of suitable employment 'without good cause'. Between 1957 and 1969 about a hundred men were prosecuted each year. In 1970 the numbers fell to fifty-eight.

The motives behind prosecution are complex. As always notions of punishment, deterrence and treatment jostle each other somewhat uncomfortably. There is no doubt that in the minds of officials prosecution may play a part in deterring others from idleness. To this end press publicity for 'successful' cases brought to court is welcomed for its potential deterrent effect in a particular area. Behind this may also be the concern of the SBC that 'justice is seen to be done' by those who readily criticise the laxness of our social security system and who resent 'the scroungers getting away with it' as it appears to them. Some of this resentment also exists within the ranks of the officials themselves. This factor may be of more importance than the deterrent effect on a particular man.

There is some, though slight, evidence concerning the impact of prosecution on individuals. A study was carried out of the subsequent work records of 360 men prosecuted between 1957 and 1961.[1] Of these 247 were imprisoned; 49 put on probation; 76 fined; and 31 conditionally discharged.

[1] Unpublished report by a civil servant as part of a programme of private study.

The success rate in terms of immediate subsequent employment appears to have been in the region of 50 per cent. The percentage of success (which is based upon rather small numbers) varied considerably according to the sentence: 45 per cent of those imprisoned; 66 per cent of those put on probation; 54 per cent of those fined; and 71 per cent of those conditionally discharged. (Courts can now impose a suspended sentence.) The reasons for these substantial differences are obscure without further study. One obvious question would be the relation of prison sentences to previous criminal records but there is no evidence on this point. However, the maximum period of imprisonment for this offence is three months, which, given remission for good conduct, means two months, and very few would claim reformative value in a short prison sentence. Indeed, in view of the overcrowded prisons and interaction of criminals, the contrary may well be the case. But of course once prosecution is initiated the matter is out of the Department's hands.

As one would expect, further analysis of the figures shows diminishing returns for second and third prosecutions, although there are some successes—which highlights the difficulties for the Department in deciding when to initiate further prosecution. There is, not surprisingly, less probability of success where there is a criminal record. There seems little to indicate greater chances of success according to whether a man was married or single, the size of his family or his age but some indication that prosecution was more effective if initiated earlier rather than later.

Such data kept in more elaborate form would be of considerable value and statistics to facilitate analysis and give guidelines for policy about prosecution are now being kept.

More recently, Headquarters staff have looked at the results of prosecutions in 1968. Some interesting points, which merit further study, emerge although the numbers are small. (Information was available on 79 out of 86 prosecuted). Of the 79, the results of prosecutions were:

Suspended prison sentence	26
Prison	19
Fine	13
Probation	10
Suspended prison sentence and fine	6
Conditional discharge	3
Dismissed	2
	——
	79

Various records were compared in the year preceding and following prosecution on leaving prison. The effect on the subsequent work record was examined for the group as a whole. (It was not, of course, possible to subdivide that in terms of different 'treatment' because of small numbers). It was clear that overall there was an improvement in work in the year after prosecution, 44·5 per cent having worked twenty-four weeks or more of that year, compared with 20 per cent the year before. However, within that average, it was found that 24 per cent worked *less* in the year following prosecution and 25·5 per cent worked for about the same length of time. Thus about half of the men studied worked substantially *more* in the year after prosecution, of whom about 25 per cent worked *considerably more*, i.e. sixteen weeks or more.

A further interesting finding was that, despite the above, there was also an increase in weeks of certified sickness in the year following prosecution: 17·5 per cent of the men were sick less: 56 per cent were sick for about the same period: 26·5 per cent were off sick more, of whom a very small number (2·5 per cent) were sick for considerably longer periods. These figures, of course, make the overall increase in numbers of days worked even more significant. It is obvious that the interpretation of such a finding is impossible without deeper study. We do not know if this is a real increase in sickness, in any way attributable to prosecution, or simply to a greater readiness to go to the doctor for 'legitimate' cover.

Clearly there are many other aspects of this problem that merit further study. Social workers would no doubt welcome a subtler kind of analysis between the characteristics of the individual men prosecuted and the results achieved. Such a study, however, has many methodological problems and it is rather doubtful whether the SBC would be justified in a costly research into an aspect of its administration that is relatively insignificant in terms of numbers, important as its consequences may be for individuals.

However, it must be a matter of concern that some of the men who are prosecuted are the least adequate of a group who evade work. The evidence needed to establish a case for prosecution must be based on a number of proven instances of refusal to take, or relinquishment of, suitable employment. Thus the 'sharper' men, with a delinquent mode of life, can often manoeuvre situations either to avoid being offered employment or to take jobs for short spells when they know the eye of authority is upon them. Furthermore they will sometimes have lucrative employment 'on the side'. Thus it seems that some of those who do eventually reach the courts are either the least adequate or those whose antagonism to authority is a mark of personality disturbance.

The papers of all men for whom prosecution is being considered are appraised by a Senior Medical Officer in the region. They may be referred for a psychiatric examination at his discretion. This does not, however, dispose of the problem: first, because the boundaries of psychiatric illness are ill-defined; secondly, because the views of medical officers about the value of psychiatric investigation for claimants of this kind may vary and in any case the boundaries of psychiatric illness are ill-defined, and third, because some man may refuse the examination. However, it must be emphasised that the papers of those men submitted for prosecution are now examined at Headquarters with meticulous care for signs of physical and mental disability or family stresses. Much depends here on the observation and recording of local office officials, which is not geared to such descriptions. Nonetheless, it is the writer's impression that few stones are left unturned that might throw light on the problem and local officials are under instructions to seek the opinions of social workers known to be involved when prosecution is contemplated. But, despite the formal controls of bureaucracy and the development of official policies there is no escaping from the effect, at higher as well as lower levels, of particular officials' responses to such cases. Thus there is need for continuous examination of prevailing attitudes.

Prosecution is regarded by the Supplementary Benefits Commission as a last resort and is in many ways an administrative gesture of desperation. It should be considered in relation to earlier measures, described earlier, taken to control the problem, and to the effectiveness of the earlier forms of intervention currently practised.

Local Office Attitudes

Thus far, special aspects of administrative policy have been discussed. However, the attitudes of non-specialist officials at field level are equally important. Unemployed men form a high proportion of those who call at the office. Because of arrangements with the Department of Employment and Productivity, they are likely to crowd the office at certain days of the week, notably Fridays. They are thus the focal point of considerable organisational difficulty and tension. They are also the focal point of much of society's ambivalence about means-tested benefits. For, as has been shown, it is exceedingly difficult, if not impossible, to distinguish between need and exploitation in certain instances. SBC officials inevitably reflect society's ambivalence. Their short basic training attempts to grapple with this in drawing their attention to the significance of their attitudes to the unemployed and the underlying problems that may exist. But it is doubtful whether such training can affect attitudes to any great extent, especially if the climate of a particular office is unsympathetic to unemployed men. The psychological (and on occasions even physical) tensions in the office situation, added to the relatively low salaries of clerical officers who interview and pay money over to the unemployed men, create in some areas a situation in which resentment by officials of such claimants seems inevitable. It seems probable that such prejudices as do exist against the unemployed man will have certain tangible effects on the claimant's well-being. It may in certain instances result in inappropriate application of the controls described earlier. However, for those men with dependents, to discontinue benefit is rarely possible and it is important to note that unemployed men receive proportionately more exceptional needs grants than do any other group, although this is to be expected as men required to register do not receive the 'long term addition'. It cannot be too strongly emphasised, however, that in any system there will be a gap between formal policy and informal organisational behaviour. Such a gap is in part created by the attitudes of officials who are individuals with feelings of their own and are given roles that are very different from those traditionally allocated to the bureaucrat. This is crucial to the understanding of the treatment of unemployed men.

Social Workers and Voluntary Unemployment

These chapters, which have been concerned with 'voluntary unemployment' have, in the writer's view, demonstrated the complexity of the problem as far as social policy and the administrative process are concerned. They offer a perfect example of problems in the exercise of a social control function—problems with which social workers in this country are currently much preoccupied in various areas of their activities. If one accepts, as the present writer does, that some such element is present whether explicitly or implicitly in almost all social work, the question arises as to whether 'voluntary unemployment' is a field of practice in which social workers ought to take more interest. It is clear that social workers' lack of involvement arises in the main from the structural division of cash services from social work. 'Rehabilitation programmes' for the unemployed have long featured prominently in some countries in which this division of service has not occurred.[1] In Great Britain social workers have specifically focused on the problem only within the Industrial Rehabilitation Units. Family Service Units and the Probation and Aftercare service have paid more attention to it than local authority services, except for individual attempts in certain areas.[2] In general, however, it is undeniable that social workers have not made this matter a focus of special concern in work with families, which has been much more centred upon mothers and children. (This may have weakened the impact of much family casework.) Clearly, if social workers do not accept the value of employment to the man and his family in those cases with which they are working they cannot press forward with conviction. It is the writer's impression, however, that many social workers do not refrain from conviction but rather because their training and allocated roles have not encouraged them to take this aspect of individual and family functioning into their frame of reference.

Once the relevance of such employment problems is accepted by social workers in particular instances, it is unarguable that they require as high a level of skill in study and treatment as any other. There appears to be no justification for a situation in which one group in the community—a number of whom present severe social and psychological problems—have had a much smaller share of time and skill focused upon these difficulties by the personal social services than others.

In saying this, one is not seeking to imply exaggerated hopes for the efficacy of social work intervention. On the contrary, as recent researches have demonstrated,[3] social workers must be increasingly cautious of making omnipotent claims. However, the understanding and treatment of the voluntarily unemployed cannot develop unless it is more closely associated with work on comparable social problems and accepted as meriting the same degree of social concern. It seems likely that, immature and uncertain as it may be, the social work profession is the right place for this to develop. But the present structural division, in addition to the current pressures on social workers and their long-standing uninvolvement with this problem makes it unlikely that, in the near future, social workers outside the Supplementary Benefits will play a significantly greater part in work with the voluntarily unemployed. However, the basic question remains

[1] For example, in Israel and the USA.
[2] For example, in the (former) Middlesex County Council where Eugene Heimler. supported by the NAB, took a keen interest in employment problems of the mentally ill, See E. Heimler, *Mental Illness and Social Work*, Penguin, Harmondsworth, 1967.
[3] For example, see Goldberg, op. cit., and Davies, op. cit.

—whether it is justifiable, especially in the light of the new unified local authority departments, to keep efforts to help the voluntarily unemployed within a service not geared to such activities. In so doing, do we simply accept that, administratively and statutorily, change is too complex to contemplate? Or do we, in fact, collude with the long-standing segregation of the unemployed man as less deserving? The development of training courses for Unemployment Review Officers and other staff concerned with voluntary unemployment centred upon educational institutions and run by social work tutors is potentially of considerable importance—as is the research (described in Appendices I and II) which is being undertaken by the Oxford University Department of Social and Administrative Studies—in bringing the complexities of the problem to the attention of social work educators and, therefore, hopefully in time to the social work profession generally.[1] The strains on social work resources at the present time need no elaboration. But in the long term it seems that greater involvement in this problem would be most advantageous in three ways: first, the claimants might benefit either directly from social work help or indirectly from social work influence on SBC policy; second, social workers' work with families and individuals will be enriched by taking this dimension into account to a much greater extent than hitherto; third, the Supplementary Benefit Commissions might be, to some extent, relieved of a time-consuming and worrying task, to which bureaucratic structures are not really suited.

[1] The Oxford social work course now includes unemployment among the social problems students may study.

CHAPTER 6

UNSUPPORTED MOTHERS[1]

This chapter examines some aspects of the Supplementary Benefits administration in relation to unsupported mothers. It does not attempt to consider their social and emotional difficulties except in so far as these bear directly on the administration of the scheme. Nor does it comment in detail on their financial circumstances since they have been studied by others[2] and are present within the terms of reference of the Finer Committee.[3] However, many of the issues raised by the discussion that follows go far beyond the confines of the Supplementary Benefits scheme and involve consideration of family law, changes in which may be essential if the situation of 'unsupported mothers' is to be improved. In general it must be emphasised that the position of such women is extremely weak. By virtue of their concern for their children and their desire to keep them, they are more vulnerable than any other group. For many, life seems just a long struggle in which there can be few of the social and personal enjoyments that women in ordinary families now expect as of right. Their financial insecurity looms large and may lead them into emotional tangles and to conflicts with the Supplementary Benefits administration. For example, the financial burden of a new baby may be a factor in a woman's decision to cohabit: contrary to her hopes, she may find herself inadequately supported and thus be tempted to deny it in order to retain her benefit. It is of the utmost importance that the extremely complicated technicalities of the law and administration should not blur the crucial matter: the extent of the difficulties and the suffering many unsupported mothers experience.

Liability of Relatives

As the term 'Liable Relative Officer' implies, the Supplementary Benefits administration is as much concerned with the men who are liable to maintain women and children as they are with the women.

---

[1] The phrase includes widows, divorcees, separated wives and unmarried mothers.
[2] See Appendix IV.
[3] Independent Committee appointed by the Secretary of State to study the problems of one-parent families under the chairmanship of Mr Morris Finer, QC.

This will not be considered in this book because during the writer's term as Social Work Adviser it was not possible to study this in depth. However, the omission is regrettable since in a sense it colludes with the tendency to consider only the women in such situations as relevant to consideration of welfare. Clearly this is not the case: the ways in which Supplementary Benefits officials approach such men; the attitudes adopted towards them; the payments reached by voluntary agreement between the SBC and the men—all these factors have significance for the wellbeing of the men concerned and possibly also repercuss on the women. For example difficulties between separated husbands and wives may be exacerbated if Supplementary Benefits contact with the man reveals to his cohabitee a situation of which she did not know the full facts. This in turn may affect a man's attitude to his wife and to their children. Officials are instructed to approach their task with tact and great emphasis is laid on confidentiality. It will readily be appreciated, however, just how sensitive some situations are and how likely it is that on occasions difficulties will arise. The official is often visiting an unknown man in a different area from that serving the woman claimant and fragmentation of roles make it difficult for the Supplementary Benefits administration to attempt to see the family situation as a whole and to relate decisions taken about finance to that situation.[1]

Numbers Claiming Supplementary Benefits

The numbers of separated and divorced women and single women with illegitimate children in receipt of Supplementary Benefit have been rising very sharply in recent years. In 1964 there were about 119,000 separated and divorced women receiving supplementary benefit; by 1970 there were 172,000. For mothers of illegitimate children,[2] the increase has been even sharper: in 1946 about 22,000 were receiving supplementary benefit. By 1970 the number had risen to 67,000. Of course this is still a very small proportion of the total receiving supplementary benefit. But this group of claimants is undoubtedly very time-consuming for the administration for a number of reasons: first, unlike the elderly who comprise about 70 per cent of the total, they tend to come off and on the books because of more frequent changes in their personal circumstances; secondly, the Commission is bound to investigate the liability of certain men to

[1] See Chapter 3 and later in this chapter.
[2] This category includes single women, separated and divorced wives, and widows.

I

maintain their dependents;[1] thirdly, suspected abuse in particularly complex circumstances must be investigated.

Reasons for Increase in Claims

The dramatic increase in the numbers of women claiming benefit, linked to a general increase in pressure of work and consequent difficulty in making thorough investigations, have combined to create mounting anxiety among staff that abuse among 'unsupported mothers' is on the increase. In fact, of course, the rise in the number of women with dependent children claiming benefit is a complex phenomenon, likely to be associated with important changes in social behaviour and deserving closer study. It seems likely that the dramatic increase in the numbers of unmarried women with children claiming supplementary benefit has some connection with the lessening of stigma, both in relation to attitudes towards illegitimacy and to the claiming of supplementary benefit. There is no certainty that a higher proportion than in the past are abusing the scheme, in the sense of claiming dishonestly.[2] However, the very existence of such a scheme plays some part in the social change that lies behind these figures. Thus for women who wish to keep their illegitimate children or to separate from their husbands, entitlement to supplementary benefit is bound to be in some cases a contributory factor in their decision, as is the Commission's policy that it will not require women with dependent children to go out to work. Furthermore the trend, which is related to changes in the social and moral climate of our time, poses problems for the Commission in the application of its cohabitation rule. As will be discussed later, the main difficulty for the Commision lies, not in defining the principle, but in the definition and interpretation of it in practice.

Problems for Policy and Impact on Officials

Such difficulties are bound up with changes in acceptable behaviour between the sexes, as for example the degree of financial support a woman expects from the man she lives with and the degree of commitment in sexual relationships. It must be acknowledged, therefore, that the increase in the number of women claiming benefit brings in its train an increase of situations in which official decisions concerning entitlement are bound up with complicated family circumstances.

---

[1] Ministry of Social Security Act, 1966, Para. 22 (i).
[2] Abuse of the Supplementary Benefits scheme is currently under investigation by the Fisher Committee, appointed in 1971 by the Secretary of State for Social Services.

As this chapter will demonstrate this group of claimants presents greater difficulties to the official than any other in the exercise of individual judgement. For many of the women straightforward financial help is all that is required and it would be inappropriate, even undesirable, to encourage officials to ponder upon the personal and domestic complications of such women. However, it seems that without some understanding of such factors, officials are likely to be preoccupied to excess with the question of abuse and may have difficulty in managing their own reactions to such claimants; for among fatherless families every kind of distress, difficulty and tragedy may be found. This is, of course, true of other groups of claimants on Supplementary Benefits. But a large number of the elderly, for example, who receive a supplementary pension are people whose only problem is financial; the same is true of a fair proportion of the temporarily unemployed. The long-term sick present, inevitably, many emotional and practical difficulties but their situation is such that they do not pose the same problems in the *administration* of the scheme as do fatherless families. Fatherless families are peculiarly 'at risk' as far as their handling by officials is concerned since their financial need is often inseparable from their personal problems and their domestic complications. Almost by definition the term 'fatherless family' implies anxiety, sorrow and sometimes tragedy at some stage. In a week's visiting from local offices the writer saw: a woman whose husband had returned unpredictably and violently to assault her and the children; two whose husbands had sexually assaulted their children; one whose husband had deserted her and the army, leaving her 'an outsider' in an army camp; an educationally subnormal girl of 17 who had just had a child; a recent widow in heavy debt; the daughter of a general practitioner whose husband was in prison following fraud; a West Indian who was suspected of 'battering' her eldest child; and a woman whose husband had become acutely mentally ill, had assaulted her, torn up bedding and burnt money. Of course not all the precipitating events were recent; people learn to adjust to past sorrows and get on with the business of living. Yet these types of situation, so commonly found, are bound to make a considerable emotional impact on the officer.

In such cases it is exceedingly difficult for the interviewing officer to find an appropriate emotional position or stance in dealing with claimants at times of distress. This is not simply a question of time: it is a question of the attitude and degree of involvement shown in the time available. Obviously this applies to the whole range of supplementary benefit work and not only to fatherless families. But it has a particular significance for fatherless families in view of the complexities of the situations that arise in this group and with which the officer must deal daily. The officers required to make decisions at field level are members of that society whose ambivalance about unsupported mothers is so marked. Thus difficulties of maintaining a sense of proportion are even greater than in some other types of case—such as those of voluntary unemployment. This is partly because detection of dishonesty does not necessarily imply that the woman are financially secure; and partly because everyone's feelings about problems concerned with sexual relationships are intense, involved, and usually little understood. By contrast, for example, the average officer's reaction to 'layabouts' is more straightforward. Thus one officer may have powerful feelings of compassion towards the forsaken wife and of antagonism to a deserting husband. Another may react harshly to women who are believed to be 'promiscuous'. These feelings have a bearing on the decisions taken. They will meet with some women whose personal relationships are difficult, disturbed and sometimes destructive; they will sometimes encounter them at times of stress and crisis when claimants' feelings are unusually intense and when the presenting need for money is bound up with the alleged desertion by a husband or cohabitee. Supplementary Benefits officers are no more exempt from reactions to those intense situations than anyone else. Thus, in an area in which judgement has to be exercised in a variety of ways that directly affect the welfare of claimants— above all in relation to the situation in which allowances may be refused, restricted or withdrawn—the existence of strong currents of feelings and the interaction of these feelings between officers and claimants must be taken in account in considering the administration of the scheme.

Negative Discretion

There can, for example, be differences in the amount of money a woman receives when she calls at the office according to whether a 'provisional' payment is made—entitlement having been established— until her circumstances have been fully verified, or whether a lower 'part' payment is made because the officer is not satisfied that entitle- ment is appropriate and abuse is suspected. Such a decision is at the discretion of the Executive Officer, but if a part payment is made and entitlement subsequently established, it should not affect the arrears she subsequently receives. To ignore the relevance of attitudes to the decisions taken is just as unrealistic as to ignore the existence of instructions on the matter. As has already been indicated,[1] the present organisation of the work and in particular the narrowness of the role allocated to the Liable Relative Officer may militate against effective concern for the social problems so frequently associated with such claimants. The reaction of officials thus interacts with their prescribed roles which may on occasion lead either to unconstructive inner conflict or to reinforcement of unhelpful attitudes.

Claimants at the Office

Reference has already been made to the problems of the physical conditions of local offices.[2] This is, of course, a matter of concern in relation to all claimants but it may be particularly distressing for some women who, at times of sudden emotional shock, find themselves in physical surroundings which they may feel to be degrading. Thus their self-respect may be diminished by such experience at the very time when it is already at a low ebb. It would be tempting to suggest that separate reception and interviewing arrangements might be made for women callers but such divisions always tend to sharpen the distinctions between 'the tough' and 'the soft' elements in the administration and would almost certainly mean that less care was taken over office conditions for the unemployed men.

It is also arguable that, in addition to the provision of private interviewing facilities, women who have young children with them should go to the head of the queue—an arrangement already followed in a few offices. The strain of waiting with fretful and noisy children is considerable and complicates life for the staff as well as for the claimants. No matter how efficient a visiting service is offered, there are always bound to be a considerable number of women calling because of sudden domestic upheavals. The treatment they receive when they call will leave an indelible impression as do, for example, similar experiences of hospitals at times of crisis, when one is particularly vulnerable. Subsequent home visits, even if sympathetic, will not undo those first vivid impressions. To some extent the writer's observations in the matter of callers confirm those of Marsden[3] that for many mothers the first encounter with 'the system' if it took place in a local office, was distressing.

[1] See Chapter 3.
[2] See Chapter 1.
[3] D. Marsden, *Mothers Alone: Poverty and the Fatherless Family*, Allen Lane, London, 1969.

The Visiting of Fatherless Families

Until recently, officials were instructed that all women with sole responsibility for dependent children should be visited every thirteen weeks, unless they were in a household where there were other active and responsible relatives who appeared to have the interests of the children at heart and where there were no outstanding welfare problems. The changes in visiting procedures, already outlined,[1] should in theory release time for more flexible and frequent visiting for those who need it most. Clearly the earlier arrangements were too rigid. For within this group of woman there is every range of competence and incompetence, financial difficulty and (relative) comfort, honesty and dishonesty. However, the old arrangements illustrate the attempt of the (then) National Assistance Board to provide a visiting service related to the welfare of claimants as well as to the problem of abuse. Nowadays one would hope that, increasingly if not yet sufficiently, such women will find their way to other social services in relation to particular problems; which makes it hard to justify the continuance of the old NAB pattern. Nevertheless, there is a strong case that claimants who fall into this category should be visited quite frequently in their first year on the books. Support could be given at the time when the claimant is most likely to need it and most likely to get into financial difficulties. Bereavement, divorce or separation are all forms of loss. They may lead to atypical unstable behaviour for a time, in which financial difficulties loom large. For some women the sheer shock of having to manage their own affairs leads to panic and anxiety and they would profit greatly from sympathetic practical advice at such a time. For others the depression, mixed with inexperience, may lead them to act foolishly—for example, taking on excessive hire purchase commitments in an attempt to cheer themselves up. A sympathetic official knowledgeable about financial matters, legal proceedings, hire purchase and all the other problems that face a woman soon after such loss, could make an invaluable contribution to 'welfare' in the period of readjustment. Similarly the unmarried mother coping with a baby in difficult conditions would often be glad of such advice and support.

'The writer visited Mrs Z, in her fifties, suddenly widowed a year ago in September 1968. Owing to waiving of visits, she was not visited between September 1968 and March 1969. The Executive Officer who visited at the end of that period found she was "at her

[1] See Chapter 3, pp. 64 ff.

wits end" with new hire purchase commitments for a three-piece suite and certain other items, all necessary but also, perhaps, a reflection of her need to bring a new brightness into the house at such a time. He was able to advise and to help financially on these matters but took the inquiry no further. She was then not visited until August 1969 when another officer, inquiring carefully about her situation, elicited the fact that she was very short of bedding and was worrying about the approach of winter. An exceptional needs grant was made. As we left the house, the woman said with an expression of relief and pleasure, "It's good to know somebody cares".'

This woman was of average intelligence with teenage children; her husband had been a bus driver in regular employment. There was no reason to suppose that she would not settle down in time to manage her own affairs with the help of her sensible children. But it is regrettable that at the point of bereavement, she was left without a visit for six months. Furthermore, such visiting would enable a more detailed assessment of the claimant's reliability and of the need for referral to other agencies. Careful work in the early stages of a claim could go some way towards controlling the generalised suspicion that arises from official anxiety about abuse. It is too early yet to say whether such developments will be possible under the new arrangements. They would have important implications for training and would indicate a willingness on the part of the Commission to concentrate more resources on a particular aspect of the welfare function.

Women Going out to work

Women who have dependent children under sixteen living with them are not required to register for employment.[1] They may, of course, take part-time work which will be taken into account in calculating their entitlement, subject to 'a disregard'. It is not official policy either to encourage or discourage this, since it must be decided by the women in the light of varied individual circumstances. Nor should pressure be brought to bear on women to take up full-time employment. This is not to say that part or full-time work would not on occasions be beneficial to the individual concerned and that satisfactory arrangements might not be made for the care of children. It is simply that such decisions, involving as they do complex individual attitudes and domestic arrangements are best left to the mothers themselves. However Marsden[2] claimed that, despite official policy,

[1] Supplementary Benefits Handbook, Para. 7. [2] Marsden, op. cit.

pressure by officials of the National Assistance Board on mothers to take work was widespread. He acknowledged that information derived solely from the mother was unreliable especially in matters in which subjective impressions are very important.

'It should be stressed that what mothers said about their experience of national assistance, and indeed the experience itself, was probably shaped by the emotional turmoil of their broken relationships, by their anxious hopes and painful needs, their preconceptions about the nature of public assistance, their pride and their feelings about how the rest of the population looked at them.'

Despite this caution, however, and the low response rate (56 per cent) from the mothers invited to participate, Marsden slips into a general condemnation of officials on this point, failing to distinguish between subjective and objective fact. In these comments, as in others concerning the mothers' relationships with NAB officials, opinion and impression sometimes appear in the guise of research. This is not to underestimate, however, the importance of the mothers' feelings about these encounters nor the difficulty in obtaining a reliable general impression of these feelings and of the actuality. Moreover, Marsden's impressions on this point are to some extent confirmed by Morris who, in her study of nearly 600 prisoner's wives, remarked, 'there appears, in some cases, to be an undue emphasis on getting wives, often with young children, to go out to work'.[1] It is probably realistic to assume that such pressure is on occasion exerted, especially when suspicion of dishonesty exists in the mind of the official or when there is a degree of personal prejudice or antagonism. But it should not be forgotten that officials may suggest work from a genuine desire to help and this may be interpreted as pressure. The stigma felt by many women in claiming supplementary benefit may make them particularly sensitive to any remarks concerning employment. In short, this issue exemplifies the problems inherent in a system that depends largely on formalised instructions in matters involving direct contact with individuals in difficult matters, in which the attitudes of officials—both in actuality and as perceived by the claimants—are relevant to the confidence felt by claimants in the scheme. The officer is not simply an automaton, a mouthpiece of Headquarters policy: in many ways he would be the poorer if he were. Yet as it stands he may be ill-equipped to play his

[1] P. Morris, *Prisoners and their Families*, Allen & Unwin, London, 1965. It is only fair to point out, however, that both Marsden & Morris were describing the situation prior to the creation of the Supplementary Benefits Commission in 1966.

role discreetly and sensitively for he is usually unaware of the complexity of the psychological and social factors involved in the apparently simple question: 'Should she go out to work?' This is a question that he may be asked or may ask himself, whatever official policy lays down.

Affiliation and Maintenance Orders and Voluntary Arrangements

The Commission's responsibilities in respect of maintenance and affiliation orders for women claiming supplementary benefit, and their obligation to protect public funds are described in the Supplementary Benefits Handbook.[1] Officials may interview women to establish whether they are willing and able to seek their own affiliation orders and separated wives to ascertain the facts concerning the separation. In either case, although particularly in the former, intimate questions may have to be asked. It is the policy of the Commission to encourage women to obtain such orders: this, it is argued, is advantageous to the claimant as well as to the SBC. Such orders will, of course, continue even if Supplementary Benefit ceases and, in the case of separated wives, it is possible that the order may be for a sum greater than the current rate of supplementary benefit. However, a number of women, especially unmarried mothers, are reluctant to start proceedings and it is easy to see that, in such cases, there may be resentment if pressure is brought by officials to do so. Thus a situation of potential conflict exists, which may be exacerbated by the fact that the SBC, regardless of the wishes of the mother, may later initiate proceedings against a husband or father to recover benefit paid to those whom he is liable to maintain or they may apply for an affiliation order. It needs little imagination to see the difficulties this may create, for example in cases in which the father of an illegitimate child is a married man and both he and the mother of his child wish it to be kept from the wife. However, there is a very considerable area of discretion in the matter of court proceedings. Furthermore the Commission are unable to take their own affiliation proceedings without the supporting evidence of the child's mother and, likewise, proceedings for the maintenance of a separated wife are seldom possible unless she is willing to give evidence for the Commission. The Commission's officials are under instructions to interview fathers 'discreetly' and will attempt to secure a voluntary payment when an order is not in force. Indeed it is remarkably rare for allegations to be made of tactless or insensitive handling of these situations. Closer scrutiny would probably reveal

[1] Supplementary Benefits Handbook, Para. 141.

that the Liable Relative Officer can avoid awkward confrontations by accepting, without too much probing, statements declaring that the whereabouts of the man concerned is unknown or that the father of an illegitimate child is not known. It is, however, regrettable if a woman is pushed to the lengths of accusing herself of promiscuity or of lying about a man's whereabouts in order to avoid legal action or unwelcome contact being made with him.

Abuse and Suspicion of Abuse

In relation to unsupported mothers, abuse is primarily concerned with undeclared earnings, fictitious or collusive desertion, or cohabitation which is denied. The application of the cohabitation rule will be considered in some detail later but some general comment about the problem as a whole is appropriate. As has already been indicated, the issue is of paramount importance in considering the welfare of father-less families since suspicion of dishonesty may effect the treatment of women claimants.

Amongst claimants generally, undeclared earning is much the 'commonest' form of abuse. All changes in circumstances are supposed to be reported. Women's part-time earnings are particularly difficult to discover because of the nature of the employment in which some may engage and there is little doubt that for many the temptation not to declare, or to declare only a part of their earnings, is very great. In this, some employers will collude. One suspects that attitudes to this form of deception are on the whole sympathetic and that society in general has constructed its own hierarchy of immorality in which the mother who is alone, but earns 'on the side', is deemed less culpable than the mother whose supplement to benefit is derived from a relationship with a man.

Fictitious or collusive desertion describes those situations in which a woman declares her husband to have deserted her but in which this is a pretence or an agreed separation. Most frequently when this occurs the husband is in fact living away from home for part or all of the week but is in touch with his wife and giving her money. There may be some couples who have developed this technique deliberately as a useful way of increasing their income. Some officials believe, however, that this is not infrequently resorted to when the couple is in debt and can think of no other way out, or when the wife is inadequately supported. It is obvious that such consideration cannot affect the obli-gation to withdraw the allowance, yet it affords another example of the complex welfare problems which may be behind abuse of the scheme.

The cohabitation rule derives from the 1966 Social Security Act[1] which provides that: 'Where a husband and wife are members of the same household their requirements and resources shall be aggregated and shall be treated as the husband's and similarly, unless there are exceptional circumstances, as regards two persons cohabiting as man and wife.' It is also stated that: 'Where, under the following provisions of this act, the requirements and resources of any person fall to be aggregated with and to be treated as those of another person that other person only shall be entitled to benefit'.

The Commission, in their paper on cohabitation[2] comment: 'The effect of these provisions, when read with Section 8 of the Act, which provides broadly that supplementary benefit cannot be paid to a person who is in full-time work, is that a woman who is cohabiting cannot, unless there are exceptional circumstances, claim benefit in her own right and therefore is debarred from receiving benefit if the man is in full-time work.' The effect of this is to ensure that a couple who live together as man and wife receive no more and no less than a married couple. The law assumes that the man with whom the woman is living has a responsibility to support her and her children. This rule poses no problem to the administration when cohabitation is admitted.

This is not to say, however, that serious problems of welfare may not arise in situations in which the cohabitee does not accept financial responsibility. The rule is clear and rigid: its administration may cause hardship, although the Act provides for special treatment 'for exceptional circumstances'. The Commission use this loophole in the last resort to provide for the children of a former union. When cohabitation is denied, complex issues arise concerned with the definition of the 'state of cohabitation' and with establishing the facts. Denial of cohabitation thus constitutes one of the thorniest problems in the administration of supplementary benefits and possibly the most difficult problem in the matter of abuse.

It is extremely difficult to establish with any precision the extent of abuse, even if there were to be intensive investigation by techniques of random sampling. A survey of the so-called 'Liable Relative' cases conducted by the NAB in 1965 resulted in the withdrawal or reduction of allowances in 11,000 cases out of 55,000 investigated: about 1 in 5. Only suspect cases were investigated and an estimate of 7 per cent of all kinds of abuse as for this group was simply derived by applying

[1] Ministry of Social Security Act, 1966, Second Schedule, Para. 3 and Section 4(2).
[2] *Cohabitation*, HMSO, 1971.

the figure of 11,000 to the total number of cases (152,000) on the books.

Of the 11,000 cases in which allowances were withdrawn or reduced, roughly 2,000 were fictitious desertion, 7,000 were cohabitation and 2,000 were other types of false statement, such as undeclared earnings and unreported lodgers. In a written parliamentary answer in December 1969, the (then) Minister stated: 'Since then there have been smaller, limited inquiries and none of these suggests that the percentage of fraud among these claimants has increased, although the number of unsupported mothers claiming benefit has risen substantially since 1965 . . . It must . . . be remembered that in this field . . . a case of fraud may often be accompanied or provoked by grave social and human problems and, indeed, not be readily separable from them.'[1] Such limited surveys can give no more than the most general indications of the extent of the problem. However, common sense suggests it would not be surprising if about one seventh of unsupported mothers were found to be technically guilty of some dishonesty, especially if that includes undeclared earnings. In fact, taking into consideration the people, their problems and the fact that abuse is often gradual and unplanned—earnings that creep up beyond the limit, relationships that turn into cohabitation, husbands who genuinely desert but return—one might predict that the figure would be higher.

Official figures about abuse will not give the flavour of the range of people and situations that are involved. Three brief examples from the writer's experience illustrate this:

'Mrs A (divorced), lived on a council estate; custody of the children had been awarded to the father; there were two illegitimate children. A large car was parked outside when we arrived: the home showed every sign of comfort, even affluence. Mrs A, of average intelligence, was wary of our visit. "Yes, I have a boyfriend; yes, he is here now in bed—do you want to see him? No, he does not live here; you can check with the air base he works nights. But he comes every day." The children showed signs of disturbance and were fostered in the evenings by Mrs A so that she could work—earning, of course, only up to the allowed limit at a public house.

There seemed little doubt that, although cohabitation and undeclared earnings could not technically be proved, Mrs A was in fact working the system very satisfactorily to her considerable financial advantage.'

[1] Hansard, December 1965.

'Mrs B (separated) was on the same estate: there were three children of school age. Suspicions of fictitious desertion had been proved in the past when her husband had been found at home in bed. At that time she had lied at first, then admitted the truth. A depressed frightened-looking woman, probably of below average intelligence, she cared well for the children; the house was sparse and well worn. "Have you heard from your husband?" "No." "Do you know where he is?" "No, I've no idea".

There seemed quite a possibility that Mrs B knew where her husband was and/or that he was returning to the home. However, when he did return he gave her little, if any, money and her supplementary benefit represented her only financial security. It would be scarcely surprising if she should lie for she was caught in a web of marital difficulty in which she was a victim of her own ambivalence about her husband and his inability to take on the normal responsibilities.'

'Mrs C was a middle-aged widow, with severe asthma; weary-looking as if life held no pleasure. It was a comfortable older-type Council house, well worn but adequate, with a row of newly laundered shirts hanging up to air. When visited in August (last visited in February), it was discovered that her twin sons had gone to work at Easter and she had not written to inform the office of this fact. As a result, there had been a substantial overpayment. Mrs C knew quite well that she was being paid in excess; she had "sinned by omission".'

These examples show in miniature the variety of person and problem which lie behind statistics about abuse. Mrs B illustrates a further dimension of the difficulty—that serious family problems may frequently exist even where abuse is confirmed.

It is extremely difficult for officials, especially at the local level, to maintain a sense of perspective about the problem, in the face of such uncertainty and ambivalence. Staff shortages and overwork have, in the writer's opinion, played a significant part in increasing official's anxiety about abuse and there is always a danger that this will react upon the claimant in various ways. First, and most difficult to assess or prove, there is the question of attitudes. If anxiety about abuse is running high, it is very likely that this will effect the attitudes of officials, towards some women claimants, whether or not they have real grounds for suspicion. In this, as in so many other spheres, training is important, both in observation and in self-awareness.[1] It is a

[1] See Chapters 2 and 3.

matter for regret that in contrast, for example, with voluntary unemployment, there has been little emphasis in training on the problem of unsupported mothers. Secondly, anxiety about abuse may affect procedures. For example, at one time, too many women, because of vague suspicions, were brought into the local offices weekly to collect payment instead of being issued with order books. This practice did little to confirm or allay suspicions and could cause considerable inconvenience, if not distress, to the claimant. (It was much disfavoured by Headquarters and should not now take place.) Thirdly, there is, of course, the possibility that suspicion actually affects the benefit received. The difference between 'part' and 'provisional' payments described earlier is one example, although, in this case, arrears should be subsequently payable. One can only speculate as to the extent to which extra discretionary grants are refused because of suspicion. Certainly it is against official policy and it is the writer's impression that it is probably uncommon if a reasonable case is made out for the extra that is needed. More subtle, however, and impossible to measure, is the extent to which suspicion may make it difficult or impossible for the claimant to ask for help or for the official to offer it unasked.

All this should not blind us to the plain fact that suspicions may be well founded, that abuse does exist and that officials are bound to be aware of this possibility in their dealings with claimants. It is simply to point out how the problem may affect interaction with claimants and that, in an exaggerated form, it has serious implications for the well-being of this group.

The Cohabitation Rule

The difficulty and importance of this aspect of the Supplementary Benefits administration is demonstrated by the Commission's decision to publish a paper on the subject, only the second of its kind.[1] In this paper the philosophy underlying the law is ably analysed and convincingly argued:

'It is not the business of the Supplementary Benefits scheme either to penalise or to favour those who are not legally married. A man who is entitled to supplementary benefit living with a woman not his wife is entitled to benefit for her, and for their children, when he is sick or unemployed: it would be manifestly unreasonable if, while he is at

---

[1] *Cohabitation*, op. cit. Three more are in preparation.

work, his partner could claim supplementary benefit for herself and children in her own right.

It has been argued that a cohabitation provision is in itself wrong; and that since cohabitation has no legal statute a couple who are cohabiting should not be dealt with in the same way as a couple who are married. Neither under the Ministry of Social Security Act nor under common law, has a man any legal liability to maintain a woman to whom is he not married (unless in the case of a divorced woman there is a Court Order), nor her children, unless he has been adjudged to be the father. He should not therefore be expected to support them in the context of the Supplementary Benefits Scheme. If the cohabitation rule were removed from the Act, the women cohabiting with a man would be treated as a claimant in her own right, any resources she obtained from the man being taken into account. It has also been argued that the cohabitation rule is out of tune with modern trends of life and that the effect of the Commission's intervention in what is essentially a private matter can be damaging to the persons concerned in other ways than the purely financial.

The Commission recognised that there has been some support for this view; and we therefore think it right to examine it in some detail. But at the same time we should like to make it clear that we do not accept that it is well founded; that we do not think there is a viable alternative to the present rule; and that we consider that in general there is public support for the present policy. In our view it would be wrong in principle to treat the women who have the support of a partner both as if they had not such support and better than if they were married. It would not be right, and we believe public opinion would not accept, that the unmarried "wife" should be able to claim benefit denied to a married woman because her husband was in full-time work. We express no opinion about whether this would be an encouragement to immorality. But it would certainly be attacked as a discouragement to marriage, as indeed in many cases it would be, since the couple would be better off on supplementary benefit than if they were married. It would create difficulties for the couples who, although not legally married, wished to be regarded and treated as though they were (especially where the marriage is invalid but one party thought it was valid). Such couples probably represent a large proportion of the numbers to whom the cohabitation rule applies. It would entail investigation into marital status in all cases. It would present an obstacle to the legitimation of children; and perhaps reverse the rise in recent years

in the number of legitimations which are shown in the figures
published by the Registrars General. And it would remove some of
the pressures on a man to support his own children.'

The paper goes on to consider the administrative difficulties that
would arise if the financial requirements of a cohabiting couple were
treated separately and points out that, since the financial arrangements
between cohabiting couples vary greatly and are difficult to ascertain,
it would be virtually impossible to arrive at an equitable assessment.
They continue:

'It would, moreover, be difficult to decide who, for supplementary
benefit purposes, had the responsibility for the children. There
would be obvious difficulties about leaving this to the claimants,
since responsibility might then be attributed in whichever way
produced the larger supplementary benefit payment: on the other
hand it would be invidious for an arbitrary view to be taken by the
Commission on who had had, in fact, the primary responsibility.
Moreover, it is also of the utmost importance to consider the effects
on the children. Divided responsibilities and disputes about responsibility could be psychologically and socially harmful. The
inherent difficulties in settling this point underline the fallacy of
pretending that the requirements of a cohabiting couple are in
essence any different from those of a married couple.'

They conclude:

'The legislation merely gives formal shape to what remains the
desire of society as a whole for fairness and equity in the distribution of the State's financial support to men and women and their
children. It contains an element of moral judgement on, or penal
sanctions against, informal unions which are not legalised. Critics of
the cohabitation rule, if they are to establish a case against it, must
demonstrate that society as a whole believe that men and women
living together but not married to each other should be given
privileges, so far as supplementary benefit is concerned, for which
married couples are not eligible.'

Within the framework of existing social and moral conventions, the
case as presented by the Commission seems unarguable. The underlying assumption, however, that a man who lives with a woman must
take financial responsibility for her and her children is one which
some would question. There is little doubt that the existence of a

sexual relationship between the couple (as distinct from sexual *relations*) is at the centre of the cohabitation issue. In contrast, if two women lived together with the children belonging to one and shared a common household, the working partner would not be expected to support the woman with children. The position is commonly misunderstood by social workers who suggest that the cohabitation rule implies a moral condemnation. This, as the Commission rightly argues, is not so. Yet, it is not correct to dismiss the existence of sexual relations between the couple concerned as only one of a number of equally important criteria in determining cohabitation. It is possible for there to be sexual relations without cohabitation: but it is rare for cohabitation to be determined unless there is a strong probability of the existence of sexual relations.[1] This represents not a moral condemnation; it simply reflects the fact that sexual relations lie at the heart of the marriage. The moral value is contained in the cohabitation rule which in essence implies that a shared household with a woman carries with it for the man a financial responsibility comparable to that of marriage. It may be that, as the Commission argues, the cohabitation rule is not 'out of tune with modern trends'. However, it is important that the values underlying such legislation should be carefully examined in the light of changing patterns of behaviour, if for no other reason than because there may well come a point when such regulations become virtually unenforceable if a section of society, men and women alike, do not subscribe to the morality underlying them. Ultimately, the law can only work by consensus.

The Problems of Applying the Principle in Practice

However, in the writer's opinion, the greatest difficulty in this matter lies not in the principle but in the application of the principle in practice. There are three main stages in determining whether cohabitation exists when it is denied. First, identifying such cases; secondly, establishing the facts; thirdly, applying the criteria to the established facts to decide whether a case has been made out.

Identification of Cases

The first stage—of identification—raises quite fundamental issues of policy concerning the zeal with which officials should pursue inquiries. Officials are under the clearest instructions that they should not approach claimants with generalised suspicion and that they should only pursue inquiries when there are grounds for suspicion. This

---

[1] The position of elderly couples in respect of this rule raises some thorny issues.

K

being said, however, it is obvious that such instructions leave a good deal to the judgement of the official as to what *are* grounds for suspicion and even more detailed official guidance cannot eliminate the need for such judgement, especially when an interview suggests the possibility of cohabitation for the first time. On such occasions the official may not follow his inquiries up and may seek approval for further investigations from a senior officer. But this will mean that occasionally an opportunity is lost for establishing the facts, especially when there is reason to believe that the claimant is inclined to dishonesty.

Many such investigations begin as a result of allegations, sometimes anonymous, received by local offices. It is the usual practice to follow these up, unless there is reason to believe that they are quite unfounded. This is an aspect of the Supplementary Benefits administration which social workers find distasteful although they also have to follow up similar allegations as, for example, of child neglect and ill-treatment. There is no doubt that many such allegations are actuated by spite. Unfortunately whatever the motive the information may be correct. It is difficult to see how it could be ignored. Indeed, in the long run, given the ambivalence about the scheme and at times excessive anxiety among the general public that it is being exploited, to ignore such allegations might work to the detriment of claimants as a whole by creating greater pressure to restrict benefits in various ways.

A similar rule to that of the sbc in relation to 'mothers alone' exists in relation to widows' benefit administered by the 'Insurance side' of the Department. These inquiries are pursued with rather less vigour than those of the sbc, which might lead to a suspicion that widows on the whole receive preferential treatment to other unsupported mothers. Against this it may be argued that the great majority of widows are elderly and that for most of them the possibility of cohabitation is remote; whereas, in the case of unsupported mothers, it is obviously numerically a much greater problem, potentially much more expensive, and more likely to attract attention from the general public. Such differences as do exist serve to illustrate that the mere existence of a rule gives no guidelines to the administration as to how rigorously it should be enforced.

Establishing the Facts

Establishing the facts regarding cohabitation is probably the most sensitive aspect of this administrative problem. The Commission acknowledge this:

'The mere fact of investigation in this emotionally charged field arouses distress and resentment among claimants, social workers and others, perhaps beyond that aroused in any other area of the Commission's administration. And establishment of the facts and their interpretation is bound to be difficult and time-consuming. Questioning about domestic circumstances where there is no acknowledged cohabitation will be resented. If a woman has been receiving supplementary benefit for herself and her children she will have an incentive to deny that she is cohabiting if this means that her allowance is withdrawn because the man is in full-time work. This will especially be so where she is unsure that he will stay with her or unsure whether he will maintain her and her children. Sometimes she will feel, however carefully questions are put to her, that moral criticism is implied; and she will resent what is, however one would wish to disguise it, an intrusion into personal privacy which is no less painful for being inescapable. Officers are reminded that, when a couple are not openly living as man and wife, special tact and discretion must be used in eliciting the facts; but what may be seen generally as tact and discretion may be viewed very differently by the claimant and indeed by workers and others concerned with the problem or consulted by the claimant.

The couple must be living in the same household. The officer may be satisfied that this is so but it may be denied; enquiries may have to be made in the neighbourhood or a watch kept on the house; the woman may say the man is only visiting; he may claim to have another address. On the other hand, where the man is simply using the house as an accommodation address, it may be difficult to prove one way or the other. Even if there is no doubt that the couple live in the same household it still has to be established that they are living together as man and wife. At this point the difficulties facing an officer are extreme, especially in cases where their relationship is neither stable and permanent nor casual and promiscuous, but something in between.'

This is commendably frank for a document of this kind and points to the essential difficulties. However the detailed problems thrown up by this basic task of investigation deserve closer examination. For they reveal the tight-rope the Commission walks, between unwarrantable intrusion into peoples' domestic and personal affairs and ineffective enforcement of the regulations. Consider, for example, the matter of visits. If it is desired to establish whether or not a man is living in the

house, an unnotified evening visit is obviously useful in some circumstances. Clearly, however, such visits can be resented as an encroach-
ment on the claimant's private life. Should observation of the house
replace evening visits wherever possible or is the former more
distasteful than the latter? If evening visits are paid—how late?
Clearly, visits after bedtime are intolerable. Is 'tea-time' better, when a
man is just home from work? In what circumstances should sleeping
arrangements be looked at? Perhaps most crucial of all, how should an
interview be conducted when it is desired to establish whether or not
cohabitation exists? To what extent is a Supplementary Benefits
official entitled to use methods of interviewing which resemble those of
the police? A further difficulty concerns procedure in relation to the
voluntary surrender of books. When an order book is voluntarily
surrendered at the time of interview, there is obviously a possibility
that it is done out of fear or anger prompted by the official's handling
of the situation. Equally, the claimant may do so because she knows
the allegation to be correct. What safeguards are necessary to avoid
'involuntary voluntary surrender' and to ensure that a woman knows
she may re-claim if she has acted impulsively? Once the principle of
investigation has been officially acknowledged, the policy-makers must
grapple with all these questions and many more; and whatever
answers they give, it is inherent in the situation that the individual
officer and the local office must still be allowed some discretion. It is
right that the Commission should point out that there are 'thousands
of cases where necessary investigations . . . have been fairly and
tactfully carried out' and this is a tribute to the British official, both at
field level and at the higher levels, much needed to balance frequently
exaggerated criticism. Equally, it is important to demonstrate just *how*
complicated the ground rules for such investigations must be: an
issue to which, it may be felt, the Commission did not give full
weight in their paper.

Application of the Criteria

A third aspect of the cohabitation rule is the application of the criteria
to the established facts in order to reach a decision.

'The Commission's officers have then to reach a judgement on
whether or not there is cohabitation on the basis of the facts of each
case. They have to take this into account, for example, whether the
couple are publicly regarded as living together as man and wife,

whether they are really sharing the same accommodation and, if so, how the household expenses are shared and what sleeping arrangements are. It is not enough to show that a man is sharing the same house—he may be a bona fide lodger. Nor is it enough that a man may visit the house from time to time and sleep with the woman. These circumstances do not constitute cohabitation.

While cohabitation has to be taken as a legal term having a precise meaning (and one common to the social security field as a whole) the basic difficulty is to determine, on the facts of any case, whether a man and woman can be said to be 'cohabitating together as man and wife' when relationships between husbands and wives vary infinitely. One aspect of the marriage relationship which is of extreme importance and might possibly, however, have been given too little emphasis in the past is the context of cohabitation. This is its public acknowledgement; the couple may have in some way indicated their status as man and wife. This may be either as open acknowledgement by them—the appearance of the same surname on the electoral register—or a previous claim of any kind by the man in which he recognised the woman as a dependent. The Commission have considered, but reject, the proposition that where there is no public acknowledgement the couple should not be considered to be living as man and wife. This would not only be illegal: in practice it would be unrealistic to treat public acknowledgement as if it were the sole test of cohabitation. To do so would, for example, put a premium on concealment.'

However, the Commission go on to agree that public acknowledgement of the union should be the first aspect to be considered. 'A rule to that effect would prevent unnecessary or premature enquiry into personal relationships and domestic arrangements.'

It is clear that when public acknowledgement is not made a judgement will have to be made on 'a balance of probabilities'. It would be ludicrous to supply officials with a 'check list'; but guidance on criteria to be applied and, to some extent, the relative weight to be given to them is obviously necessary. One of the most difficult issues concerns the amount of time a man may spend in the same household before he becomes a 'cohabitee'. And what if he has a wife somewhere else, with whom he lives part of the time? The possibilities of fatuity in regulations and the inevitability of their arbitrariness if any consistency between cases is to be achieved, is obvious.

Welfare Responsibility

The problem does not, however, end for the Supplementary Benefits administration when a cohabitation decision has been taken. The Commission's formal welfare responsibility remains. It is not uncommon for there to be financial hardship as a result of the decision, more especially in cases where there are children of a former union which the man is unwilling or unable to support. The Commission 'reject the proposition that . . . supplementary benefit should be paid as a matter of course to the cohabiting mother for all her children who were not of the current union'.[1] They point out that this would act as a disincentive to marriage and place such couples in a better position than those who are married. Nevertheless they concede that 'in the last resort' they would pay benefit for the children 'where they would otherwise suffer hardship or where the refusal of benefit might mean the break up of the household to the detriment, for example, of any children of the current union'.[2] This is a neat illustration of the tension between proportional and creative justice which has been referred to earlier. The argument against preferential treatment for the unmarried is unanswerable. Equally, the humane policies of the Commission ensure that they would not wish ultimately to be responsible for the break-up of an individual family. It is, in the opinion of the writer, greatly to the credit of the Commission that they have made a public acknowledgement of this important area of discretion. However, it is clear that, in practice, such situations are likely to produce considerable tension between officials on the one hand and claimants or social workers on the other. The official has the phrase 'as a last resort' in the foremost of his mind. How is he to judge whether this point has been reached? On what criteria? Whose word is he to take? Such cases also involve consideration of the local authorities' discretionary powers under the Social Services Act 1970 to help certain families by direct financial assistance. The Commission has re-affirmed its responsibility for welfare *referral* in such cases, when children are involved.[3] This should not be seen as an evasion of financial responsibility by the SBC for the children of such unions since it is obvious that many such situations will need social work help in addition to, or instead of, financial support. Furthermore, it is important for the field staff of the SBC that this has been publicly stated because there has been a tendency to overlook the family difficulties of those detected in abuse of the scheme. Nevertheless,

---

[1] *Cohabitation,* op. cit., Para. 31.   [2] Ibid., para. 32.   [3] Ibid., para. 33.

referral may on occasion be, or may be seen to be, 'passing the finan-cial buck'. This is inevitable and derives from the present confusion of responsibility, and the practical difficulties of interpreting 'the last resort'.

The Commission comments that 'critics of the system sometimes complain that evidence obtained in this way is acted upon though it would not stand up in a court of law'.[1]

'This shows a fundamental misunderstanding . . . [Inquiries] are not intended to be automatically a preliminary to a prosecution for which, in any case, the evidence must be such as to establish guilt beyond any reasonable doubt. They are intended to discover facts on which to make a judgement about the case as a whole. This will include a decision as to whether, on the balance of probabilities, cohabitation is shown—a judgement which can be challenged forthwith in an informal appeal tribunal.'

In contrast with other sections of the paper in which these thorny issues are very fully explained and discussed, the treatment of this important point seems somewhat cursory. Behind it lies the important distinction between the burden of proof necessary to establish entitle-ment as compared with that needed for a prosecution. If these processes were to be confused, one unfortunate outcome might be that in cases of disputed cohabitation, there would be pressure to prosecute unsuccess-ful appellants. This is of general relevance to the field of social security, for example, in the payment of contributions. Nevertheless, the distinction leaves the door open to maladministration, simply because 'the balance of probabilities' rests—quite inevitably—on the judgement of officials rather than on more clear-cut evidence.

This, of course raises the further question of appeals in such cases. How effective a safeguard is the possibility of appeal bearing in mind the sort of claimants involved and the difficulties involved in the voluntary surrender of order books? Behind such questions lies the more fundamental issue of the value of legal or quasi-legal procedures in ensuring justice for claimants—an issue explored by Titmuss,[2] who is scathing about the American enthusiasm for lawyers. He rightly points out that 'the belief that lawyer's law contains no element of discretion is completely false. Law and discretion are not separated by a sharp line but by overlapping zones'. The same, of course, applies to

[1] *Cohabitation*, op. cit., para. 23.
[2] R. Titmuss, 'Welfare Rights: Law and Discretion', *The Political Quarterly*, Vol. 42, No. 2, April 1971.

Appeal Tribunals whose decision on matters of cohabitation would inevitably involve judgements 'on the balance of probabilities', as do those of officialdom. It could, however, be argued that a greater degree of impartiality could reasonably be expected from such Tribunals and that it might therefore be appropriate, not only to encourage appeals, but to evolve some machinery whereby such decisions were, as a matter of course, taken by some independent body; at the very least such procedures would act as a brake on the administration. However, such a policy would inevitably raise many other questions. How many other areas of discretion should be vested in an independent body (for example, decisions on cases of fictitious desertion)? How does the selection of tribunal members safeguard objectivity? Does its quasi-legal standing effect a successful compromise with regard to the nature of evidence? Most important of all, can any such structure deal effectively with the imprecisions and subtleties of a cohabitation decision, any more than it can deal with the intricacies of a parent–foster parent dispute over a child?

Any consideration of the present system raises the important issue of the levels in the hierarchy at which decisions should be taken, whether they are decisions to pursue investigations, to assess the balance of probabilities, or to take specific action following the withdrawal of benefit, such as welfare referral. The seriousness with which these decisions are viewed is witnessed by the fact that there has been a tendency of late to pass responsibility 'up the line' to senior officials in local offices. This is welcome, not necessarily because the senior official is better equipped to decide on individual cases—though this may be the case—but because, within a bureaucratic system, such a procedure automatically emphasises to officials the importance of the matter and increases the probability of objective decisions, insofar as these are possible in such a complicated matter.

Thus we have seen that the justification for the cohabitation rule must be examined in the context of the techniques needed to establish the facts and the validity of the criteria adopted to define it. Difficult as it may be to find just alternatives—and this has been admirably argued in the Commission's paper—the changing nature of roles between men and women and the extreme difficulty in practice of defining the term to cover the infinite variety in such relationships leads one to doubt whether the rule in its present form can be indefinitely sustained. It is not surprising that Executive Officers, far from being over-zealous, are frequently disinclined to probe too far.

Conclusion

The role of the Supplementary Benefits Commission in relation to 'mothers alone' affords a useful illustration of some 'diswelfares' resulting from the complexity of administrative practice and organisation; most of them result from the basic principle in our society concerning responsibility for maintenance. Whilst there may on occasions be officials who, as individuals, demonstrate excessive zeal or prejudice, the welfare of claimants will in the long term be better served by examining this principle and the administrative structures which have developed to implement it than by pillorying individuals. Certainly, the problems of the Supplementary Benefits administration must be seen in the context of the provisions of the social security system as a whole for this group. The findings of the Fisher Committee will be eagerly awaited. So far as the Supplementary Benefits scheme is concerned, reorganisation and better training of staff would go some way towards meeting the problem. Yet, as long as the principle of 'liable relative' responsibility remains in its present form, there will be a degree of tension between the statutory responsibility of the SBC to ensure that the liable relative assumes his responsibilities and the need to protect claimants and liable relatives from excessive inteference with their private lives.

However, it must be borne in mind that, of the unsupported mothers receiving a supplementary allowance, 'liable relative' problems arise in only a proportion. Many women effect satisfactory financial arrangements with husbands and fathers. Many require only reliable financial service. For them, the present machinery of the SBC works quite well, especially when an order book has been issued and they need have no direct contact with the local office. Apart from the possibility of a more supportive service in the early stages of their 'aloneness', there is little more that could be done for them within the Supplementary Benefits scheme as it stands—that is to say, without considering more radical changes in the method of financial support for mothers alone. Why then focus so much attention on the few—perhaps not more than two or three per cent of the total receiving supplementary benefits? The answer is twofold: first, because this book is concerned with minorities, believing that this is the proper concern of social work; second, there is no doubt that the total group of unsupported mothers would be at risk if concern about 'liable relative' responsibility were to become the dominant feature of the administration.

CHAPTER 7

SPECIAL WELFARE OFFICERS

This chapter will describe in detail the work of the Special Welfare Officers within the Supplementary Benefits Commission and will analyse some of the issues and problems that arise from such a description.[1]

The work has been outlined briefly in Chapter 3 in which certain categories of cases were suggested in order to give an idea of the kind of problem that comes the way of the s w os. Such a categorisation is, however, incomplete and at this stage more precise information is appropriate.

Referrals to Special Welfare Officers

In the quarter from 1 May 1969 to 31 July 1969, 441 cases were accepted for action by s w os. The people concerned were receiving supplementary benefit for the following reasons:

	No.	%
Over pension age	76	17·2
Incapacitated by sickness or injury	109	24·7
Fatherless families	149	33·8
Unemployed	85	5·0
Unable to work because caring for other person(s)	22	19·3
	441	100·0

In these 441 cases, 1,041 specific problems were identified. These were connected with:

	No.	%
Mental disorder	167	16·0
Mismanagement of money	342	32·9
Self-neglect	90	8·6
Physical handicaps	32	3·1
Ill health	104	10·0
Accomodation	41	3·9
Unemployment	83	8·0
Sickness at home or loss of wife	24	2·3
Problems of unmarried mothers	14	1·3
Problems of widows and deserted wives	134	12·9
Others	10	1·0
	1,041	100·0

[1] The training of s w os is discussed in Chapter 8.

The 167 cases of mental disorder and the 342 cases of mismanagement of money were distributed as follows:

	Mental disorder	No. of cases Mismanagement of money	Both categories*
People who were:			
Old	38	51	76
Sick	73	82	109
Unemployed	34	54	85
Responsible for fatherless families	19	148	149
Looking after some other person	3	17	22

*The two groups overlap.

There is no reason to suppose that this sample is not representative of the usual pattern of referrals. The figures speak for themselves and to a social worker the probable complexity of many of the situations behind the figures, especially in relation to the high proportion of mentally disordered persons in the sample, is self-evident.

Development of the Specialisation

Special Welfare Officers were first used in 1961 when three were appointed on an experimental basis. Since then the numbers have crept up, most regions having at present four or five. Although their numbers are small their very existence is, in principle, of great importance since it demonstrates the difficulty the Commission has had in safeguarding its 'welfare functions' without some form of specialisation within the organisation. Furthermore, this arose at the very time when other social work services, especially in the local authority, were developing apace. Paradoxically, such developments may have indirectly contributed to this expansion, first, because there is more awareness in society generally of the need for such services; secondly, because of the increased pressure in relation to welfare by the social work profession on the Supplementary Benefits administration. The growth of such a specialisation within the SBC, however, gave rise to anxiety within the administration. This anxiety revolved around two questions. To what extent was there inappropriate overlap with the existing social work services? To what extent would any further development prejudice the development of social work services outside, especially in the local authorities? The Seebohm Committee discussed this issue briefly:

'It has been suggested to us that there would be advantages in giving officers of the Supplementary Benefits Commission responsibility for carrying out some welfare work with their own clients in certain circumstances. We are aware that in present circumstances it is not always easy for the Commission's officers to know with certainty which services would be appropriate for particular clients. Officers sometimes feel that, after referring a case, the action that follows is tardy and inadequate and that sometimes there is no action at all. Moreover, in some circumstances, the Commission's officers may feel that their own responsibility is inextricably involved and they may wish to work closely with the service to which the client has been referred.'

Despite these arguments the Committees were crisp in their recommendations:

'It seems to us that a natural and helpful division of responsibility emerges between the Commission and the new Social Service Department . . . *We consider that the Commission's officers should refer cases to that department and should not attempt to undertake social work themselves.*' (My italics)[1]

The superficiality of such a statement is understandable since their terms of reference did not require them to consider the workings of the SBC. However, an analysis of the work of the SWOS is probably the most effective way of demonstrating the difficulties in applying in practice such a deceptively simple principle. It also serves to draw the attention of social work readers to the existence of the SWOS. It appeared during inquiries that few social workers knew them. Those who did welcomed them in somewhat vague terms. Clearly, however, the implications of such a group, however small, for future policy is of considerable importance and the defining of the boundaries of their work and of their roles should be of concern to the social work profession.

The following description arises from the writer's study of the work of Special Welfare Officers in 1968. Of course, since then there have been changes, including those consequent upon the recommendations made. In essence, however, the problems and the tasks remain the same.

At the time of the study, the work of the SWOS fell into one of three categories. First, there were those functions which, it will be argued, are 'permanent and indispensable', that is to say, those which a means-tested scheme of this kind may always require if it is to

---

[1] Report of the Committee on Local Authority and Allied Personal Social Services, Cmd. 3703, 1968, Paras 684, 685.

administer benefits with due regard to welfare. Secondly, there were those functions which were necessary at that time to the administration because outside social work services or the general work of the SBC was inadequate. Thirdly, there were those functions that were not, strictly speaking, relevant to the administration of supplementary benefits and in which the referral had been prompted by a more general concern for the welfare of claimants.

Permanent and Indispensible Functions
1 Mental Disorder

The high proportion of the mentally disordered on the caseload of the SWO has already been noted. The term is used with some precision: that is to say, most of the individuals thus described would fall into the conventional, clinically recognisable, categories of mental illness.[1] There is no question of marking down any claimant who is a nuisance to the SBC as 'mentally disordered'. On the basis of the writer's examination of all case-papers from one region over a period of three months and of discussions with twenty SWOs and regional staff, there emerged the strongest evidence that many of the claimants thus described were only marginally able to cope with life in the community and would doubtless in other days have been in hospital.

This observation raises the question of the adequacy of community services for the mentally ill. However it would be naive to suppose that improvements in such services would obviate the need for specialist intervention within the SBC in certain cases. This is because, for some people, money matters can become the focus of intense disturbance and result in a sense of grievance for alleged injustices or excessive demands for extra financial help resulting from acute anxiety.

This is not to underestimate the real difficulties people may have in making ends meet; nor to overlook the fact that mistakes and injustices in the part of the Supplementary Benefits administration do occur. The group of claimants under consideration, however, are those for whom everything possible within the rules and regulations governing the scheme has been done. Before their papers reach a Special Welfare Officer, they have always been the subject of special consideration at local offices and have often been referred to regional offices for advice. Despite all efforts, however, their difficulties and their grievances persist. Their disturbance is focused on the Supple-

---

[1] The writer does not intend, in this context, to enter into the 'labelling' dispute (cf. Goffman et al.) of which she is, however, aware.

mentary Benefits administration which cannot ignore complaints or requests but whose officials may be baffled as to what to do. Furthermore, referral of such problems to a local authority social worker may not be effective since the claimant may reject such an intervention, preferring direct contact with the officials who control the financial resources. Until the formation of the new local authority departments, there was the additional problem that the mentally disordered might be fearful of, and reject contact with, social workers to whom the labels of 'mental welfare' were attached. It will be interesting to see if this changes. But it is probable that even with the advent of a social service department there will be some who refuse to acknowledge any problem except the immediate financial one and who will not therefore accept the attention of a social worker, even if available. For others the process of such referral and acceptance may be protracted—a point to be discussed later—and the Supplementary Benefits administration may have to work towards such a referral over a lengthy period.

'An example of a claimant with a grievance is Mrs A. Mrs A. is 50 years of age. She has been in receipt of supplementary benefit since 1960, having spent the three previous years in a mental hospital. From the records she would appear to be severely disturbed but since 1960 she has not been considered sufficiently ill to warrant in-patient treatment and she rejects the Mental Welfare Officer. The s w o took on this case because Mrs A's sense of grievance and persecution resulted in constant appeals, letters and objections, including frequent visits and communications to the regional office. Her complaints were most throroughly investigated but it was found that her entitlement was being full met. Before the s w o took over there were fifty-two recorded conversations (by phone or visit) with her over a period of about two years in which many different officers were involved. Twenty-two visits were paid in one year. It was hoped that steady and quite frequent visits from one person would help Mrs A to contain her grievances and would make her feel safer than had her previous disconnected contacts.'

These difficulties also arise in relation to another group of the mentally disordered who concern the Supplementary Benefits administration because they are living below subsistance level. They usually fall into one of two categories. Some are failing to claim what is their due, perhaps because of a refusal either to register for work or to obtain a doctor's certificate. Such claimants do not usually demand attention. On the contrary, they are usually reticent. Yet the concept of entitlement, linked to a statutory responsibility for welfare, makes it inevitable that the Commission should be concerned when such difficulties are uncovered.

Mr and Mrs B and their twin children, boys of 17, were referred to the swo because the children in the household were not working and had not done so since leaving school. They refused to register for work or to attend a doctor. The family situation was revealed to be exceedingly disturbed and it is probable that both children were schizophrenic. The children never left the house. They flatly refused to cooperate with various people who had made efforts to get them into work. There is little doubt that, had allowances been withdrawn, four would have lived for the price of two. The family were not in debt and were not a trouble to any other social service.'

The Special Welfare Officer in this case had a dual function. So long as there are rules concerning procedure before benefit is payable, somebody has to deal with the casualties of the system, who are unable to cope and who will require careful handling if the situation is not to be made worse. But, additionally, the swo had a delicate task in leading such claimants to seek appropriate help from a doctor or mental welfare department. It is hardly necessary to emphasise that this is a delicate matter as the following extract from the swo's record illustrates:

'Considerable time was spent at the house. The boys would not come from their bedroom where they had locked themselves in. Parents stated that the Welfare Officer had called to see them the previous day and it had been suggested that they be seen by a doctor. Several attempts were made to speak to them through the door but they would not reply. I said I would make a further visit on another day to be arranged.

The Mental Welfare Officer expressed the opinion that we (i.e. the sbc) might be able to establish a relationship, especially in view of his bringing in the medical advice which the family obviously resent. Through the payment of allowances we have already made a big breakthrough and he would be grateful if this relationship could be maintained.'

The second group of mentally disordered claimants living below subsistence level are those whose financial affairs are in confusion and who have debts. Frequently, the picture such claimants present of their financial affairs is vague and muddled, fact and fantasy being interwoven. The official whose task is to establish facts beyond reasonable doubt in order to determine entitlement may find himself baffled. To ascertain the facts may be a complicated and time-consuming process, although one which, because of the financial need, is urgent. To introduce a social worker from another agency at this point might be inappropriate and unacceptable.

'Miss C is 62 and has been known to the Department since December 1966. The case was referred to the s w o in August 1968 because of the confusion in her financial affairs and the fact that she "had been calling at the Area Office, taking up considerable staff time but making little sense in her statements." Between August 1968 and January 1969, when the claimant was admitted to mental hospital under an order, the s w o paid fifteen visits and there are recorded contacts with twenty-eight other persons, including friends, banks, the Electricity Board and the Mental Health Department, in connection with the problem.'

The extracts from the case-papers which follow are given in some detail to convey some of the problems confronting the s w o in face to face contact with such claimants.

'Most of the afternoon with the claimant I merely contented myself with listening to her story of her much better past and in scrutinising a mass of papers, particularly legal correspondence, which she produced. The latter proved interesting but unfortunately not very revealing. Most of this was in connection with legal action which she took against a builder who undertook alterations for her to her present home. (The conveyance sighted today.) The purchase price was £3,250 which had been advanced by a solicitor friend pending sale of other house. This was supposed to have been disposed of eventually for £5,000 or £7,000 but I could get no clear picture of this or the disposal of any balance due to her. The background is very vague and sketchy here which is very unfortunate as I have a feeling that there is considerably more to this case. In many ways the home here and this woman gives an impression of affluence in the past and yet the picture now is of extensive debt, not assets, and an attempt to clear her accounts from a limited income of pension and supplement.

The debts so far uncovered are as follows: electricity £100 including court fees and solicitor's charges. The supply was disconnected last year and county court action taken to recover the debt—an order for £2 per calendar month was made. SEGAS—details unknown but she pays 40p per week. Post Office Telephones—details unknown but she pays 50p per week when she can. Rates—outstanding, account not known, pays 10p per week when she can. On this basis she is trying to pay approximately £2 per week off her debts out of her limited income which is clearly ridiculous. She lives a spartan existence and most of her life seems to be spent in the kitchen.

Not an easy person to interview, seems to have difficulty in concentrating and throughout our discussion today she kept losing her train of thought. On occasions when she went upstairs to search for various documents I could hear her talking away to herself and I formed a general impression of her being rather more than eccentric.

Contact with Local Authority: During the course of their dealings with this woman they came to the conclusion that she was mentally ill and in need of treatment. G.P.'s were contacted but little progress was made. In social worker's opinion this woman needs to be examined by a psychiatrist *but she will not, of course, cooperate.'*

The Special Welfare Officer records that some twelve months after the initial referral the claimant was admitted to a mental hospital under Section 29 of the Mental Health Act (1959) (a three day order) and that an extension of the order was to be sought. However, this had only been precipitated by a physical deterioration in Miss C's condition and the SWO had taken the initiative in contacting the Mental Welfare Officer. In other words, the SWO had conducted a holding operation, arising from concern over the claimant's financial confusion and consequent extreme poverty.

It is, of course, possible that more effective mental health social work services could have reached such people as have been described above. Yet, in the light of what is known of the importance of motivation in accepting or refusing social work help, and the anxiety for some in acknowledging mental disturbance, it seems extremely likely that for a proportion, at any rate, of those described, the SBC is in a better position to attempt to gain their confidence. However, *this contact is central to the primary task of the Supplementary Benefits scheme: that is to say, such claimants could only be disregarded if the statutory obligation to have regard for welfare were to be ignored.*

As has been said, obviously not all claimants with serious financial problems are mentally disordered. Nor is it intended to suggest that

L

they form more than a small minority of supplementary benefits claimants. They certainly do, however, form a high proportion of those referred to swos.

II Other Claimants in Financial Difficulties

Some others who get into financial difficulty may do so because of inadequate resources. It is widely recognised that social workers have been called upon to paper over the cracks of basic poverty arising from inequalities in the structure of our society and that, on occasion, they have colluded with this. No doubt the same charges can be levelled against Special Welfare Officers who are even more closely identified with the system that employs them. Without in any way underestimating the importance of such observations the fact remains that there are those whose difficulties arise, wholly or in part, from some form of social or personal inadequacy. This is no news to social workers but tends in the present climate to be an unpopular view. It may be a long-standing problem or it may occur temporarily as a result of a traumatic event such as the death of a partner. In the former cases, social work services are or should be involved. In the latter, this is more arguable; at such a time the Supplementary Benefits administration may have an important part to play in a short-term contact.

Clearly, in cases of people whose financial difficulties are chronic and part of a complicated interaction of factors—economic, social and psychological—the role of the swo must depend on the availability of help from other sources. However, it is important to consider whether some form of specialist within the sbc would be necessary whatever the resources available from other social services. One of the central difficulties in relation to such claimants concerns the exercise of discretionary powers, in particular to make 'exceptional needs' grants. This particular group of claimants brings into sharp focus the issues discussed in Chapter 2. Among them are a number whose material and financial needs are both urgent and recurring yet their use of what is provided, including discretionary grants, appears wasteful. As has been discussed in detail, to decide what kind of liaison between social work and income maintenance services would be most effective in relation to the exercise of discretion is both difficult and controversial. Certainly the Special Welfare Officer specialisation cannot be justified on these grounds alone. In fact, a specially designated official within a local office might be more effective in performing such functions than an swo since the regionally-based swo is at times viewed somewhat suspiciously by local offices as being excessively generous in discretionary grants. (There is, in fact, no firm evidence that in general swo intervention brings more money to claimants.) This may affect local relations with social workers and, in turn, their clients. However, the fact that such a role is often performed by swos at present, indicates that in the present structure the need exists for a person inside the system to examine requests for discretionary help with some degree of specialised understanding of the individual's problem so that cash assistance may be related in these instances to an overall plan for constructive long-term help.

The following is an example in which an swo was not involved. (It might have been advantageous if one had been.) The story is given in detail to illustrate the complexity of the discretionary decisions which have to be made in a minority of cases and the exceedingly time-consuming liaison required.

Mrs Long was rehoused in a local authority flat from a hostel for the homeless on 15 July 1968 and moved into this area. She had no furniture at all. The Executive Officer, Mr Bridge, and the Welfare Officer, Miss Young, cooperated to try to settle Mrs Long in her new home. (The Welfare Department were involved in their role of resettling homeless persons, and had guaranteed the rent for the new flat for two years.) In February 1969 Mrs Long was taken to court by the Education Authority because June, her daughter, had not been going to school and the Court made an order for the Children's Department to supervise June, since when Miss Hampshire has been dealing with the case. Events since July 1968 as recorded in the Supplementary Benefit case-paper were as follows:

1. Called at previous area office before 15 July 1968 to ask for grant for linoleum and curtains to move into new flat. Given £17. Did not move into flat. Went to stay with mother.

2. *22 July.* Visit by Mr Bridge (all subsequent visits were made by Mr Bridge) to mother's flat. Mrs Long said she could not move to her new flat—no furniture. Mr Bridge arranged for WRVS[1] to supply and deliver furniture. Delivery date arranged but Mrs Long did not turn up, and furniture taken back. Grant of £1 10s to WRVS for transport charges. Order-book issued for £10 13s a week—as if Mrs Long at new address—allowing rent £4.

3. *22 August.* (*a*) Telephoned Miss Young regarding non-delivery of furniture. Miss Young had arranged holiday for Mrs Long and June

[1] Women's Royal Voluntary Services.

beginning 24 August. (*b*) Visit to Mrs Long—no explanation for not turning up for delivery of furniture. Matter to be left until return from holiday.

4. *26 August.* Telephoned Miss Young to arrange further date for delivery of furniture. Miss Young said she would supervise this. Subsequently two beds and mattresses, a table, four chairs and one easy chair delivered and grant of £7 paid to WRVS for delivery charges. Claimant moved in early September. Nothing further until:

5. *14 October.* Housing Department telephoned to say arrears of rent £42.

6. *17 October.* (*a*) Visit. Miss Young said rent not paid because buying things for flat. Still had no floor covering or curtains— spent £17 given in July on other things (not known what). Told she would be paid rent weekly at Area Office. Order-book issued for £6 13s and balance of £4 to be paid weekly at Area Office. (*b*) Telephoned Miss Young to inform her of this. (*c*) Found June not going to school—telephoned Education Department about this. They said they had difficulty in contacting Mrs Long.

7. *6 November.* Request from Mrs Long for help to obtain kitchen table and chairs.

8. *12 November.* (*a*) Visit. Arranged for WRVS to supply kitchen table and chairs (grant of £3 for delivery charges). Noted June still not going to school and condition of flat deteriorating. Advised Mrs Long 'to take more interest in child and home'. (*b*) Telephoned Miss Young to report all this.

9. *4 December.* Mrs Long called at Area Office to request more furniture. WRVS driver had said that other people got more. Wanted a wardrobe and rugs, and help with heating. (Nothing done about this.)

10. *16 January 1969.* Miss Young telephoned to say case conference to be arranged. Asked if rent could be paid direct to Housing Department—Mrs Long had not paid rent for months. She had not been calling at Area Office to get balance of allowance—this had gone unnoticed by office. Mr Bridge said he would look into this.

11. *17 January.* Visit. Mrs Long had not been paying rent as dog had chewed rent book. June at school. Flat in a mess—dog had gnawed

furniture. Mrs Long wanted to start work part-time. (No further mention of this.)

12. *21 January.* Miss Young telephoned. Rent arrears over £60—eviction being considered.

13. *31 January.* Case conference.
Main points:

(a) Eviction proceedings in Court, 4 March 1969, if arrears not paid in meantime. £72 owing.

(b) Furnishing of flat. Miss Young and Mr Bridge to visit together to see what necessary.

14. *5 February.* Visit regarding request for clothing for June for her to go to school. Grant £11 15s given.

15. *7 February.* Visit with Miss Young. Arranged as follows:

(a) Miss Young to arrange for two new armchairs to be delivered and old ones to be taken away.

(b) Miss Young to arrange with Housing Department for repairs to June's bedroom—very damp.

(c) Coalmen to deliver 3 cwt. of coal—Mr Bridge agreed to give grant.

(d) Mr Bridge to arrange for floor covering.

(e) WRVS to be asked to supply more furniture—particularly chest of drawers.

16. *10 February.* Visit to get information about floor covering needed.

17. *13 February.* Mrs Long called at Area Office. Bought Wellingtons for June. Needed fares to attend Court. £2 given.

18. *21 February.* (a) Mrs Long called at Area Office with coal bill. Given £2 19s. (b) Telephoned Miss Young to inform her of this. She said two armchairs had been delivered. Court hearing regarding June adjourned. Mr Bridge asked if charitable grant could be obtained for floor covering—Miss Young thought not. (c) Telephoned suppliers regarding floor covering.

19. *27 February.* Mrs Long called at Area Office—saw Mr Bridge. Had bought curtains, electric fire, crockery and ornaments for £1 from someone who was moving. Grant of £1 given.

20. *3 March.* Housing Department telephoned about rent arrears.

Mr Bridge said some arrears (i.e. amount due to Mrs Long) would be paid. He thought Miss Young would pay balance.

21. *10 March*. Mrs Long called at Area Office to see Mr Bridge. Worried about Court judgement that she must pay £105 rent arrears. Re-assured.

22. *14 March*. Mrs Long called at Area Office, lost 30s in street. Given £1.

23. *17 March*. (*a*) Cheque for £40 14s 9d for arrears of rent (amount not paid to Mrs Long) sent to Housing Department. (*b*) Cheque £24 12s 9d sent to firm to supply floor covering. (*c*) Note to Manager to ask for authority to pay rent direct.

24. *3 April*. Submitted to Rent Officer regarding payment of rent direct. R.O. agreed 8 April 1969.'

Such an example illustrates vividly the protracted difficulty into which some claimants may get. Those claimants who get into temporary difficulties as a result of traumatic events may not need nor want social work intervention but, in certain cases, the complications of their financial circumstances are such as to suggest the need for patient attention to unravel the knots. The Supplementary Benefits official in his role as SWO may be particularly well placed to offer such help, having certain knowledge and expertise in such matters, for example in relation to hire purchase debts.

In the foregoing discussion, the focal point of the intervention by the Special Welfare Officer has been a financial problem which cannot or should not be ignored by the SBC. The specialist, it has been argued, has a contribution to make in one of three ways: first, by long-term support and containment of claimants who cannot relate to social work services; secondly, by acting as the liaison officer between social workers and the local office in cases of special difficulty; thirdly, by investigations of short-term financial crises with remedial action and/or subsequent referral.

The SWO and the Unemployed Man

Any consideration of what have been described as the 'inescapable' functions of a specialist such as the Special Welfare Officer within the administration, must take into account certain other problems that are not necessarily focused on the financial problems—real or alleged—of the claimant. These concern situations in which the Supplementary Benefits administration has to make judgements that affect the welfare of claimants and are for the most part concerned with problems of unemployment or cases in which the honesty of the claimant is in doubt. The effect of the existence of an Unemployment Review Officer specialisation used to be that few unemployed claimants were channelled to Special Welfare Officers. The s w o was unlikely to be used in cases where the claimant was required to register for work.[1] Within the s b c there was, and perhaps still is in lesser degree, a tendency to stereotype these two specialisations as 'tough' and 'soft', although the reality is far more complex, taking into consideration the personalities of the individuals involved. However it is noticeable that a higher proportion of unemployed men are now referred to s w os than previously. Most of them are those whose wives have left home or are ill and who are looking after young children. There is also a smaller group of single men, perceived by local office staff to be strange or inadequate, often living with their mothers. Although it is appropriate that such cases should be referred to the s w o, it is clear that the local office referral is usually made in the hope and expectation that the s w o will find some way of getting the man back into work. This is understandable in the light of the statutory responsibilities of the s b c and may be in the best interests of the individual. On the other hand, it may, in certain instances, be both impracticable and undesirable, especially when the man is looking after his family. The s w o is on occasion aware of organisational pressure whatever the Commission's policy may be. He may feel that, in the eyes of his colleagues, he has failed in his handling of the case if, in the light of the man's abilities, the local employment situation, the practicalities of alternative arrangements for his children and the needs of the family, he finds that the man can not or should not go to work.

The SWO and Abuse

At present, s w os are excluded from taking on cases in which there is suspected fraud or abuse which might lead to prosecution until this has been cleared one way or another. It is felt, probably rightly, that the s w o should not be asked to combine 'a welfare' and 'a detective' function. Furthermore, in cases in which criminal proceedings are possible, there are always technical problems about any form of 'welfare intervention'—similar, for example, to those that arise for social workers when allegations of a sexual nature are made against persons by children in care. However, in some situations, especially in the case of 'fatherless families', the abuse may be inextricably bound up

[1] See Chapter 4.

with complicated personal circumstances. Thus, for example, fictitious desertion (in which the woman declares her husband to have left when he has not), or cohabitation which is denied, may in some cases arise from financial problems. The man in question may be in heavy debt or may not give his wife enough to live on. Clearly, therefore, there are some difficulties in which the early intervention of an swo might prove helpful. This rarely happens: one must ask whether this specialist is used as fully as would be desirable in relation to this aspect of the Supplementary Benefits administration.

Special Welfare Officers, therefore, at present help claimants with a variety of financial problems; such referrals fall fairly and squarely within the primary task of the organisation. It seems that such interventions by specialists within the Supplementary Benefits scheme will continue to be necessary as long as the present separation between cash and services exists, even when social work services outside are more fully developed than at present. There are also certain problems, mainly in relation to 'unemployed men' and suspected abuse which pose problems for the swo and in which he has not been used as fully as would be desirable. This is in part due to the way the work is presently organised and to technical complications but, behind this, one can detect a certain ambivalence about the treatment of claimants whose difficulties present themselves in antisocial forms.

Dispensable Functions

Not infrequently claimants are referred by the local offices to swos because of the manifest inadequacy of the local social work services to cope with the problem.

'Mr and Mrs E, a couple in their late 60s, were referred by an Executive Officer "because he is disabled, and she is having problems with shopping, etc., because of ulcerated varicose veins". The couple lived at the top of a steep hill, two miles from the nearest village. On arrival, Mrs E immediately drew the swo into her troubles, obviously in urgent need of someone to talk to. It transpired that her husband is totally paralysed from the waist down. Mrs E's immediate problem was this: she was finding it increasingly difficult to move her husband from his chair to bed and to the lavatory. Efforts to get a wheelchair had failed because it seemed to be necessary to go to the hospital first and this her husband refused to do. This practical request was, of course, only the tip of an iceberg. Mrs E had lived under a heavy strain for years. Her doctor was not helpful, calling only every three months to sign the medical certificates. No doubt further visits would reveal other difficulties in this tragic situation which is, of course, a "community care" problem in which health and welfare services should be actively involved. No such services were being provided.'

Once an swo became involved, it would not be surprising if such a case took up a good deal of time. However there was no problem that affected the sbc directly and officers are now under instructions to refuse such referrals. Nevertheless it will be many years before the social work services offer adequate services over the country as a whole and it is therefore more than likely that informal referrals to swos will in fact continue to take place, especially in areas where the local office lacks confidence in its local social work services. Furthermore once a referral has been accepted and a need established, it is, of course, extremely difficult, if not impossible, for an swo to turn his back on the problem. Yet on occasion its diffuse, subtle and long-term nature—outside the normal range of an Executive Officer's experience —makes the swo hesitant in his handling of it, sometimes reluctant to give it up but unsure of his objectives. There may also on occasion be a tendency to visit where it would be better to leave this to social workers already involved, as in the case of claimants who tend to spread their troubles around or to play people off against each other. It was the writer's impression, nevertheless, that gaps in social work provision were more often the reason for the swos intervention in situations in which the difficulties were not primarily financial. This was often the case, as has been implied earlier, with mentally disordered claimants referred to the swo. However this is not always simply because the resources of mental health services are inadequate. There is also a problem of the definition of the need for such services. Naturally enough, a Supplementary Benefits official visiting a claimant whose mental condition is extremely disturbed is likely to think that 'something' ought to be done. It is not always appreciated that if the claimant is causing no damage to himself or to others and is not motivated to receive help, there may be little that ought to be or can be done. This applies also to situations in which the condition, physical or mental, of elderly people is deteriorating but has not yet reached the point at which an order should be made to remove them from their home. At such times social work services may be relatively powerless to help and may be forced to play 'a waiting game' until the inevitable crisis occurs. If these difficulties are not understood the Supplementary

Benefits officials may turn to their own specialist for help, believing that their referral to outside social work services is unsatisfactory. Such discontent may, of course, on occasion be wholly justified; at other times, it may arise from a misunderstanding of the social work role in certain situations.

Referral to, and Liaison with, Local Offices and Social Workers

The foregoing discussion raises the crucial issue of referral and liaison, both between local offices and the swos within the sbc, and between the swo and the outside social work services.

Reference has been made to a certain insecurity and tension that exists on occasion between local offices and Special Welfare Officers. It was the writer's impression that this sometimes led to a reluctance to refuse 'submissions' (as they are called) from local offices to regional offices for the Special Welfare Officer's intervention lest this lead to disenchantment with the scheme. Such submissions are considered by an official senior to the swo who has responsibility for general oversight of the work but who is not professionally qualified. The decision as to which are suitable cases for swo intervention—whether before or after further investigation by swos—is a complicated one, turning on particular aspects of the case and, to some extent, on the realities of current local social work provision. This is one reason for the introduction of 'a social work element' at regional levels—a decision that has been approved in principle by the sbc.[1] It is also clear that appropriate referral and liaison with outside agencies requires clarification of the nature of the difficulty by Supplementary Benefits officials and for communication of the reasons for action—or inaction—by social workers following such referrals. At present the swo may be a 'linkman' between the social work services and the local offices.

The Role of the Special Welfare Officer

Many of the difficulties inherent in the swo scheme, as it has been up to now, arise from the attempt to graft a professional activity into a bureaucratic structure without the benefit of the skills, experience and training which such activity would merit. As has been shown, swos handle cases which, in their practical, social and psychological complexity, are among the most difficult in social work. The impression gained by the writer was that they were, by and large, no better and no worse than the large numbers of untrained social workers in other agencies although they are undoubtedly at a disadvantage by reason of

[1] See Chapters 3 and 9.

their isolation from the mainstream of social work activity. Like most untrained workers, they have lacked the framework of knowledge which would lead them to ask relevant questions concerning the meaning of problem behaviour and to plan in the light of the probable answers. Yet their concern and patience was evident: they were able to create and sustain relationships and were purposeful in these, except when the goals were ill-defined. Their relationships with other social workers were generally good which is of considerable importance, bearing in mind the overall situation between the SBC and social workers.

There was no doubt that many swos enjoyed the job and experience satisfaction beyond what they expected and what they had experienced as Executive Officers in local offices. They enjoyed the continuity of contact, the chance to see something through and to see results in many cases. Despite the considerable strains, therefore, and the 'professional' isolation, morale did not appear to be low. This has important implications for the administration of the Supplementary Benefits scheme. For the official who is required to administer the scheme in a humane fashion with due regard to welfare is more likely to do so if he feels involved in the outcome of his actions and has the opportunity to see people and their problems in greater depth. Regrettably, however, this is in conflict with certain other trends which, in the interests of greater organisational efficiency, limit such involvement.

This discussion, examining in some detail the operations of a specialist group who are numerically insignificant, has highlighted three areas of considerable significance for the scheme as a whole. First, it has been shown that the Supplementary Benefits administration has discovered a need for such intervention in order to perform *its own* functions adequately with due regard to welfare. Secondly, the swos illustrate that this need is not solely due to deficiencies in other services but that the relationships between those systems providing cash or those providing services require some bridging arrangements. Thirdly, the importance of this small group as a symbol of concern for welfare within the SBC should not be underestimated, particularly in relation to local office staff whose belief in the sincerity of their seniors is enhanced more by deeds than by instructions.

CHAPTER 8

SELECTION, ATTITUDES AND
TRAINING OF STAFF[1]

Most of this chapter will be concerned with the training of Supplementary Benefits staff and with investigating the extent of the impact that such training may have on staff attitudes and the ways in which its impact may be strengthened or diminished by administrative practices.

Selection of Officials for Supplementary Benefits Work
Thus far much emphasis has been laid on the effect of role expectation and, on occasion, of role conflict on the attitudes of the official. It would be naive, however, to stress this to the exclusion of the personal and individual traits that also have a bearing on attitudes although, in the opinion of the writer, such explanations have tripped too readily off the tongues of social workers. The method by which officials enter the Supplementary Benefits Commission is relevant to such considerations. On entering the civil service, new recruits in the executive grade are given an opportunity to express preferences for a particular department or ministry. There is, however, no guarantee that their preference will be granted. In former days it was unusual for a new entrant to select work with the National Assistance Board. Nowadays, he may choose, and be accepted for, the Department of Health and Social Security but will not necessarily be choosing to work in the SBC. If he knows about it at all, the hard—at times distasteful—work and the conditions of local offices may make the prospect of employment in the SBC unattractive. Certainly it carries neither glamour nor prestige. Those who are enthusiastic may be social workers *manqué* who subsequently find the constraints of the job frustrating. On the other hand the unenthusiastic recruit may sometimes find unexpected rewards in work which carries so much more human interest than is usual in the civil service. It is doubtful, therefore, whether recruitment

[1] Throughout this chapter the phrase 'human relations training' has been used to describe those aspects of Supplementary Benefits training that are not technical and that are intended to increase an official's awareness of claimants as people and to facilitate their interaction with them. It is not a felicitous phrase but it is convenient shorthand and familiar jargon in the Supplementary Benefits administration.

to the SBC should be by expression of preference only, unless the civil service were to provide much fuller information about the nature of the work than at present is available to the new executive recruit. Nor would it be right to assume that such arbitrariness in selection of staff for this type of work is necessarily unsatisfactory. Alternative methods would have to be tried to test this. It is obvious that some Executive Officers find they have skills and interests they did not know they possessed. Furthermore, the creation of the larger Ministry of Social Security and subsequently its merger with the Ministry of Health do afford opportunities for transfer within the Department to work of a different kind when an official is patently unsuited to SBC work. (This does not happen easily or frequently, however, staff shortages within the SBC make such transfers improbable in the early stages of an Executive Officer's career.)

As was indicated in Chapter 3, Clerical Officers may not fall into the general category of 'career civil servants'. Some seek employment locally and their decision to work with the SBC may be a matter of convenience. As with Executive Officers, the work may arouse their interest. But their involvement in the job and therefore the degree of their motivation for training may in some cases be lower than that of Executive Officers.

Social workers, accustomed to thinking in terms of a strong vocational commitment as essential in the choice of their career, tend to react with surprise and displeasure when confronted with the facts about recruitment to the SBC. It is clear, however, that to extrapolate from social work to the supplementary benefits scene is misleading. The social worker's task is not analogous with that of the official; the degree of involvement and the kinds of skill required are in general very different. Nevertheless the analysis of the tasks in the foregoing chapters clearly demonstrates that the work of Executive and Clerical Officers in the SBC differs from that of most other civil servants in several ways; first, in the degree of direct contact with the public; secondly, in the extent to which such direct contact is with people in acute or chronic personal difficulty or distress; thirdly (in the case of Executive Officers particularly), in the extent to which the officer's judgement of people affects discretionary decisions. Thus the orthodox bureaucratic ideal of a civil servant—whose personal attributes can be controlled by powerful role constraints, whose major virtue is believed to consist in objective, equitable application of rules—is not adequate to describe a good SBC official although it is a part of the story—a fact which social workers are inclined to overlook. In the following discussion of training it is important to remind ourselves that the additional attributes needed to perform the supplementary benefits task well cannot be *created* by training—only elicited and encouraged. It may be, therefore, that attempts to improve training without efforts to refine selection are wasteful. However, it is clear that changes in selection procedure are likely to be difficult to achieve; first, because of the uncertainty as to what alternatives would succeed better; secondly, because such changes would cut across long-established traditions in civil service procedures.

Role Conflict

Nor can training resolve problems created by the organisational structures when these put officials into situations that are intolerably stressful or in which role conflict is acute. One of the difficulties in any large organisation is that change and development do not proceed at an even pace between their different aspects. It is possible, therefore, that improvements in training may generate anxiety and even antagon-ism towards the hierarchy if it is felt that the task is defined by the trainers in ways impossible to achieve within the current structure. This problem is one with which social work educators will be familiar but is of particular importance in relation to inservice training in human relations within the sbc. For, as has been shown, roles have been structured in ways that make the application of interpersonal understanding difficult.

Challenging Authority

Anxiety and antagonism towards the hierarchy may, of course, on occasion be conducive to change. In this context, however, the inherent authoritarianism of the civil service must be recognised, for this is a factor of the utmost importance in consideration of training programmes. The effect of a bureaucratic structure is to mute criticism and to make more difficult any educational programme that aims at modifying attitudes, rather than simply at imparting information. The problem is made more acute by the brake on promotion chances which conformity may be felt to impose. This is not to suggest that officials within the sbc are not vocal in their criticisms of their own organisa-tion. But where there is not an alternative professional frame of reference nor the same degree of mobility in employment as exists, for example, between different local authorities, the desire and oppor-tunities for any strong protest or rebellion are limited. Further, the very choice of the civil service as a career may itself indicate a relatively conforming personality. The danger in so far as 'human relations' teaching is concerned is that outward conformity masks unresolved problems in attitudes to claimants that may be revealed under working conditions.

Staff Development

The effectiveness of programmes of 'staff training' may ultimately depend on subsequent programmes of 'staff development' in creating a climate in which consideration of interpersonal relations between official and claimant can thrive. Such a notion implies a continuous process in which opportunities are afforded for individual growth, whereas inservice training may become an activity encapsulated in time, place and objectives from the life of the organisation. The idea of staff development, of ongoing educational opportunities provided in a variety of ways and at all levels of the organisation is not one with which the SBC, or indeed any branch of the civil service, as yet feels comfortable. Certainly within the SBC there is a basic uncertainty as to what constitutes 'relevance' to the work and is therefore justifiable. This is well illustrated by the fact that social security officials, although officially encouraged by payment of expenses to attend extramural courses in social studies and human relations, must do so in their own time.

The aim of all staff development is ultimately to influence the members of the organisation to carry out the work in the way in which the more senior members think desirable. It is a formalised process of socialisation. The phrase is necessarily a vague one since the aims of the programmes may be promoted in a variety of ways: a few examples would be staff meetings, library facilities, seminars, or attendance at conferences. However the scope and methods of such staff development must vary greatly according to the nature of that work. The more the work to be done is affected by the attitudes, knowledge and skill of the persons performing it, the more far-reaching the programmes of staff development may have to be and therefore the more difficult the decisions as to 'relevance'. It is fair to say that at present the Supplementary Benefits scheme makes less use of such possibilities than does social work and that the definition of 'relevance' is a narrower one. This is not surprising since emphasis upon staff development is closely linked to the professional aspirations of social work. Furthermore, as earlier discussion has shown, there has been considerable confusion as to the extent and range of the know-

ledge and specialisation required to perform various roles within the
SBC effectively.

Yet the importance of staff development programmes for Supplementary Benefit officials is perhaps more easily demonstrated than for
certain other branches of the civil service, simply because the element
of personal response and initiative is greater. For such officials, high
morale and enthusiasm is crucial, not only in ensuring appropriate
attitudes to claimants but in the efficiency and equity of financial
assessments and discretionary decisions. Staff development may play
as important part in this as do codes and circulars. Furthermore, the
knowledge explosion in the social sciences and the rapid rate of
change in the personal social services will mean that an intelligent
official has a need for, and a right to, information about such developments as have a bearing on his work. Only in this way will the 'closed
system' be converted into an 'open system' in which ideas, knowledge
and constructive questioning are allowed to flow freely into the
organisation. So far, the most important element of staff development
for SBC officials lies in the provision of courses in human relations and
the social services by extramural departments and comparable institutions. Between 1953 and 1969 about 8,500 officers attended social
studies courses. Between 1958 and 1969 about 2,600 officers went to
comparable human relations courses. In 1970, 414 and 372 officers
attended social studies and human relations courses respectively—a
sharp rise proportionately in the latter.

Resistance to Change

In all aspects of education and training within the SBC, attitudes to
authority and to change—at all levels in the hierarchy—are crucial. It
is well known that resistance to change is often most apparent at lower
levels in organisations and the SBC is no exception. This raises particular difficulties in organisations of this kind which are highly structured
and in which authority is clearly defined. Change, if 'prescribed' by
higher authority, must be accepted, yet it may be resented. Such
resentment can affect the implementation of change in various ways
and nowhere is this more obvious than in the more subtle areas of
attitudes and discretionary powers. Much staff development and
training takes place at the local level and, as will be discussed later,
this level is the most powerful source of influence on staff. It may be
that the characteristic 'style' of instruction in the civil service has not
been conducive to the degree of challenge upon which the genuine
learning resulting in changed attitudes must rest. For in the matters

with which we are concerned, obedience and conformity do not of themselves suffice.

It is interesting to consider whether the challenge to established authority, at present so evident in society generally, will affect the traditional modes of instruction in the civil service; whether, for example, younger staff will openly question authority which is embodied in instructions and regulations in a way that would have been unthinkable to an earlier generation. If such a situation does arise, and these questionings are not met by open and full discussion of some decisions and policies, resentment will mount, morale will deteriorate, and there is a risk that the more energetic and adventurous will leave the service.

Technical Training

In considering these matters, however, the importance of a tradition of efficient technical instruction must not be underestimated, as it might be by those readers who come to the subject from a social worker's viewpoint. The emphasis of this book has been upon those aspects of the Supplementary Benefits scheme that are not amenable to precise rules and regulations. However, much depends on the capacity to investigate financial circumstances accurately, to establish entitlement and to make correct assessments. No amount of 'human relations' training or staff development can obviate the need for instruction on such matters. In fact, one of the problems in the scheme as it stands is that fairness between individuals is achieved at the cost of very considerable complexity in the regulations. Consequently the staff are confronted with a bewildering array of instructions concerning factors to be taken into account in reaching an assessment. The much simplified Supplementary Benefits Handbook gives only the barest indication of the technical task that must be performed and to which a considerable amount of training time must be devoted. The SBC has been rightly concerned about the effect that poor technical work would have upon claimants. The effort that has gone into improvements has included the use of programmed learning techniques which may make possible a better use of the time spent in direct contact with instructors. The success of practical and technical training can be measured more precisely than training concerned with attitudes and understanding people. It would thus be easy for the less tangible elements in 'human relations' training to be squeezed out in a battle of priorities. However this is not at present evident: on the contrary, more time has been allocated to it in recent years. The NAB accepted the

M

principle of 'human relations training' in basic courses for Executive and Clerical Officers, but the time given was small in relation to the total course. The SBC have redressed this balance and have thus reaffirmed the importance of those aspects of the work in which technical efficiency will not alone suffice. While this would be generally welcomed as an indication of the good faith of the SBC in its attempt to improve the quality of its service to claimants, evaluation of the effectiveness of such efforts is crucial. For just as in social work education much has been taken for granted and little has been tested, so there is a danger that some of these assumptions will be carried over from social work into Supplementary Benefits training.

Training for Individual Initiative

The training problems for the Supplementary Benefits Commission are inherent in the nature of the scheme, in which entitlement and discretionary powers—both negative and positive—jostle somewhat uneasily.[1] It has always been the policy that these discretionary powers should be exercised at the lowest possible level in order to avoid the rigidity and delay characteristic of many bureaucratic structures. Yet, to quote Bendix: 'The problem of bureaucracy lies . . . in the manner in which technical and administrative rationality are combined with the exercise of individual initiative in the accomplishment of a common task.'[2] This chapter, therefore, considers the training requirements for 'the exercise of individual initiative' in relation to a scheme which, necessarily and properly, takes much account of the variation in individual circumstances. It is the writer's contention that such training is of profound importance for the administration of the scheme and that, if it were not sufficiently valued within the various levels of the organization, we would see a gradual deterioration of relations between officers and their claimants and between officers and those who protest on behalf of claimants. The training relates to certain knowledge, understanding and skill which enables the individual officer to perform his task with greater efficiency and humanity.

Human Relations Knowledge

The knowledge required is concerned with those aspects of people's behaviour that have a direct impact or bearing on the officer's work. Some of it is generally applicable, such as people's reaction to stress or

---

[1] See Chapter 2.
[2] R. Bendix, 'Bureaucracy: The Problem and its Setting', *American Sociological Review*, Vol. 12, 1947.

anxiety; some of it can be related to the particular groups of people with whom officers are concerned as, for example, the elderly, the sick, the unemployed and the separated, widowed or divorced wife. Such knowledge involves consideration not only of the individual but of his family and of the social structure in which the individual or family lives.

Human Relations Understanding

The word 'understanding' implies a process in which the heart joins the head to give emotional conviction to knowledge. It follows, therefore, that genuine understanding involves sympathy and concern and is bound up with attitudes. This cannot be acquired from books or from lectures. Knowledge can be extremely helpful in the development of understanding; but understanding grows best through informed discussion with suitable people of the actual live experience of the officer in certain situations. Thus it is possible to impart knowledge concerning the background culture of immigrants which will undoubtedly diminish prejudice to some extent, as will knowledge about the processes involved in prejudice, such as 'scapegoating'. But a deeper understanding will result from an officer's reflection on his reaction to a certain individual at a certain time and he will need help to reflect constructively upon this.

Skills in Human Relations

The skills required are concerned with powers of observation, constructive listening, sensitive interviewing, distinguishing between facts and impressions, and with patterning them into a coherent shape. Here again, although certain essentials can be taught as knowledge, these skills are best developed through the day-to-day use of practice as part of the training programme.

The need for such training arises from the ways in which the British Supplementary Benefits scheme has developed. The official is in many ways a hybrid—a cross between a social worker and a bureaucrat. Some may argue that the offspring of this union is unhealthy. This may be so. But the alternatives—examined earlier in this book—also carry with them grave disadvantages. If we must simply do the best we can with our 'hybrid', training is one important element in directing and developing his capabilities.

The Concept of Training

The concept of 'training' within bureaucratic organisations must not be confused with professional-style education such as that offered to social workers by independent educational institutions. Training is more limited in scope and in time and much more narrowly job-focused. One of the difficulties in the training of Supplementary Benefits staff in any aspect of human relations is, therefore, to select and present material in a short time—the 'job implications' of which are obvious—whilst avoiding gross or distorting oversimplication. In recent years the SBC have given much painstaking thought to the development of such training and by Supplementary Benefits standards a substantially increased share of the total time and resources available for training has been given to those aspects of the work that bear directly on human relations. To outsiders, however, especially those with a professional orientation, it may still seem pitifully small in relation to the depth and complexity of the issues involved. These differences in perception should be borne in mind when, as in the Commission's recent paper on cohabitation, references are made to 'intensive training'.[1]

The Training of Executive and Clerical Officers

Executive Officers have a thirteen week tutelage period including a central course which, since 1971, has been extended from three to four weeks. The first three weeks take place towards the end of the tutelage period, the fourth week about six months after entry. The amount of time spent on human relations has thereby been increased. Clerical Officers have a three week course at the end of a ten week tutelage period. For both, the first period is spent in the local office.

All officers attend a week's Refresher Course after two years of service. These are organised at regional training centres, as are a variety of short specialist courses, for receptionists for example. In addition, for some years, central training centres ran courses for Liable Relative Officers. Since 1968, specialist courses for Special Welfare Officers, Unemployment Review Officers, and Senior Reception Centre staff have been initiated or expanded and, at the time of writing, nearly all such staff have attended them. Development of training for Clerical Officers and Assistants in Reception Centres is under way.

There are approximately 6,000 Executive and 10,000 Clerical Officers in post. All the indications are that a high level of wastage in both grades can be expected,[2] with a consequent high level of recruit-

---

[1] *Cohabitation*, HMSO, 1971.
[2] Unless unemployment should radically alter the situation.

ment, even without overall increases in complement. A survey was carried out, for the years 1962 to 1966, for young officers of both grades in the (then) Ministry of Pensions and National Insurance from which it appeared that their average service life was not more than five years. The overall wastage in the NAB during these years, expressed as a percentage of staff in post at the beginning of each year, was about 5 per cent for Executive Officers and 7 per cent for Clerical Officers. This average does not, of course, reflect the high turnover among younger staff, especially women (the long service of a few distorts the picture). Thus the task for the trainers is of considerable magnitude. In 1970 523 Executive Officers and 1996 Clerical Officers received their basic training in central courses. The overall size of the training task has a number of implications; first, organisation is complex and time-consuming and, inevitably, change becomes more difficult. Minor timetable or curriculum revision, let alone major alterations, become difficult to achieve; secondly, the fact of wastage is the strongest possible argument in favour of effective training, for 'learning on the job' is a slow business and training affords short cuts to efficiency; thirdly and paradoxically, however, the wastage may be a factor in limiting the amount of training provided, for the civil service, like a business organisation, thinks in terms of 'value for money'. This is particularly relevant in those subtler aspects of human relations training where value cannot be easily measured or related to increased efficiency. This is a real barrier to the development of secondment to outside institutions for further education.

'Human relations' education, and any form of internal specialised training, is also restricted by the deeply entrenched notion of 'transferable expertise' which has so long been a basic tenet of the civil service. This leads to a reluctance to invest too much time in training an official for a task he may leave within a few years in the normal course of his career. This tendency is likely to increase now that a large unified Department of Health and Social Security has been created. Indeed, it is thought desirable that a young official on the road to promotion should gain varied experience, especially between the supplementary benefit and national insurance aspects of the work. This is little affected by the Fulton recommendations which suggested only the broadest division between civil servants in 'economic' or 'social services' ministries. The main issues arising from the idea of 'transferable expertise' are outside the scope of this book but their inhibiting effects on training developments are clear, not only because of the fear of wasted training but also because of the assumptions that lie behind them of the civil servants' repertoire of native skills, equal to all occasions, including those which confront him in the supplementary benefits context. There is a widely held view, inside and outside the SBC, that every man can be an expert in human relations.

Staff Attitudes to Training

It is only to be expected that staff attitudes towards the 'human relations' aspects of training will be ambivalent in the light of all that has so far been described of the roles and tasks they are called upon to perform and the ways in which they find themselves joining the ranks of the SBC. However this ambivalence, as has been shown, is complex and does not stem alone from uncertainty as to the need and value of this particular training but also from the traditional ethos of the civil service. Members of the Commission are unequivocal in their enthusiasm for training—which is hardly surprising given the fact that half of them are academics. During the writer's period as Social Work Adviser, their enthusiasm was, in the main, shared by officials at the higher levels, who were nonetheless inevitably constrained by the overall policies and attitudes of the service. Central course instructors who had for a number of years been involved in such training and who had all worked in the National Assistance or Supplementary Benefits schemes were, in general, welcoming of, and receptive to, new ideas. Regional training centres had not up to that time been much involved in this type of training. Their attitudes were uncertain and in part reflected a more general problem to be found also among officials who had moved either to managerial posts in Supplementary Benefits or to 'integrated' offices from the National Insurance side. Those without direct field level experience of Supplementary Benefits work and with substantial experience in National Insurance tended to be sceptical of the need for training of this kind, which was in many ways totally alien to their perception of the effective performance of the bureaucratic task. For them technical efficiency, procedural precision and impersonal application of rules were the ends to which training should be directed. At the highest levels in the SBC, officials without supplementary benefits experience were capable of persuasion by argument. At the field level, the reality of the differences between Supplementary Benefits and National Insruance work confronted the official with the need for some special help. The scepticism, therefore, was most marked in the middle ranks, especially in regional office staff or newly promoted Managers who had not 'seen it with their own eyes'.

In local offices, attitudes to such training are determined to a considerable extent by the views of the Manager and by the norms of the group. This is of great importance in considering the impact of central courses on new entrants, bearing in mind that the first weeks are spent in the local office. This will be considered later in relation to local office training. As in so many other aspects of Supplementary Benefits work, effective training depends on a reasonable congruence between official and unofficial attitudes.

Central Training

During the writer's period as Social Work Adviser, a small survey was carried out of the attitudes of Executive Officers and Clerical Officers to their central training. One object was to find out which elements in their course they had valued most and to what extent these agreed with their perception of the qualities most important for successful work. A questionnaire was sent to 119 new entrant Executive Officers and to 100 Clerical Officers, selected at random, who had passed through one of the training centres between 1967 and 1968. Replies were received from 59 per cent of the Executive Officers and 62 per cent of the Clerical Officers—a low response rate which affects the reliability of the results. Nevertheless the replies gave some interesting information which merits further examination.

At the time when the new entrants were receiving their training the main content of the human relations teaching was contained in sessions entitled 'dealing with people'. Of course such material also came into sessions on visiting, callers, and so on.[1] But it was, in the main, separated from more detailed technical instruction. It was, therefore, possible to ask officers to place in rank order (1–10), first, their remembrance of, and second, their preference for the sessions they had been given—preference being defined as those most helpful to them in performing their duties. The main point of interest to emerge was the striking difference between Executive and Clerical Officers in the ranking assigned to 'dealing with people'. For Executive Officers it ranked eighth and ninth respectively out of ten. For Clerical Officers, it ranked third on both questions. A further question asked whether they felt that any of the sessions or topics listed had been especially helpful in increasing their understanding or skill in coping with claimants. 73 per cent of the Executive Officers replied 'Yes'. The rank order placed 'visiting' first and 'dealing with people' second. A higher

[1] The sessions combined technical and human relations content, focused specifically on the task.

proportion (89 per cent) of Clerical Officers replied 'Yes' and their rank order placed 'dealing with people' first.

This difference in response between Executive Officers and Clerical Officers to sessions specifically designed to improve understanding of, and attitudes to, claimants deserves closer scrutiny. The instructors were the same; the brief broadly the same. The foregoing chapters have shown that it is the Executive Officer rather than the Clerical Officer upon whom the main burden of responsibility for decisions rests, in particular those involving discretion. At first glance, therefore, it would seem likely that he would welcome such sessions. A possible explanation is that it is just because the burden of decision-making rests so heavily upon the new entrant Executive Officer that he is preoccupied with mastering technicalities at this stage, almost to the exclusion of subtler issues. The Clerical Officer, by contrast, may have energy to spare for such excursions into the realms of human behaviour without such a definite job focus. Another explanation might be related to the greater numbers of women among the Clerical Officers. However, the fact that a Clerical Officer remembers and enjoys them and says he finds them helpful does not of course prove that work is thereby improved. It is possible that such sessions were viewed as welcome light relief from the weight of technical instructions and that the Clerical Officer was not as anxious as the Executive Officer about time thought to be wasted: whatever the reasons may have been for the response, it lent weight to a plan subsequently implemented, to integrate this material more closely into the main body of instruction.

In an attempt to relate attitudes towards training to the priority that officers gave to certain personal qualities, these were divided into 'softer', 'tougher', or 'neutral'—the last being the commonly accepted virtue of the impersonal bureaucrat. Officers were asked to rank these qualities which emerged in the following order:

Executive Officers	*Clerical Officers*
1. Interest in people (softer)	1. Efficiency (neutral)
2. Efficiency (neutral)	2. Interest in people (softer)
3. Fairness (neutral)	3. Patience (softer)
4. Patience (softer)	4. Fairness (neutral)
5. Reliability (neutral)	5. Reliability (neutral)
6. Firmness (tougher)	6. Firmness (tougher)
7. Shrewdness (tougher)	7. Shrewdness (tougher)
8. Sympathy (softer)	8. Sympathy (softer)
9. Toughness (tougher)	9. Toughness (tougher)

In both groups, then, the 'tougher' qualities came low on the list, with 'toughness' put last by more or less every officer. Even 'shrewdness', which one might have expected to be seen by a substantial proportion as a desirable quality, is well down the list. Once again it is not possible to infer from these responses anything about the qualities that predominate in day-to-day work; nor even that the responses given were genuine. What emerges, however, is that of those who responded (about 60 per cent) they either believed authority placed a higher priority on the 'softer' or neutral qualities or they themselves believed it, or both. Even allowing for the fact that non-respondents might have answered this particular question differently, the response gives a slight indication of some prevailing attitudes. This was confirmed by the response to a further question given to Executive Officers but not to Clerical Officers: 'In handling individual cases, a choice sometimes has to be made between safeguarding public funds and ensuring the welfare of individuals. Do you think your training course laid more emphasis on one than the other?' Forty-five replied 'Yes'; twenty-three 'No'. Of the forty-five, forty-four thought the emphasis had been on welfare and nearly all agreed with the emphasis.

Some tests were made of the internal consistency of the responses to certain questions. As assumption was made that certain sessions could, as could some qualities, be defined as predominantly 'softer' or 'tougher'. Thus, for example, sessions, on 'dealing with people' and 'visiting' could be described as 'softer' whereas 'fraud' and 'liable relative' sessions were 'tougher'. Thy hypothesis was that there would be internal consistency in the individual official's view of desirable qualities and useful sessions. The results showed a very high degree of consistency (92 per cent) in the responses of Executive Officers but a much lower consistency among Clerical Officers (44 per cent). This difference was, in the main, between the value placed upon 'dealing with people' sessions and the value placed on 'neutrality' as a desirable quality. One can only speculate as to the reason for the inconsistency in Clerical Officers' responses. Perhaps this value given to neutral qualities reflects their view of what is expected of them by the system and the smaller opportunities, in comparison with most Executive Officers, for continuity of relationship with people. The high ranking awarded to 'dealing with people' by the majority of Clerical Officers, however, and the fact that the inconsistency was not as between 'tough' and 'soft' suggests that some may feel a certain conflict between their natural inclinations and what they assume is required of them in their job.

The findings of this survey have been reported in some detail in the full recognition that it can have little statistical significance since the numbers are so small and the response rate so low. Its importance lies in the questions it raises about the 'consumer' view of central training and the relation between 'desirable qualities' and training. In particular, the differences between Executive and Clerical Officers would warrant further study. The implications for the SBC for further evaluation of training in terms of 'consumer' reactions are considerable, a point to be stressed in the light of its somewhat authoritarian structure. For human relations training, if it is to have any impact, requires a high degree of participation, dependent on the congruence of the teaching with the prescribed roles, as perceived by the official.

The Context of Training

In the short period of three weeks, of which only a proportion can be devoted to human relations training and to other aspects of the social services as a whole relevant to welfare, the educational problem is one of focus and selection. During the writer's period as Social Work Adviser, a guide was produced to a 'knowledge base' for Executive and Clerical Officers, which aimed at the selection of material of direct relevance to the task to be performed. This guide covered the following:

Reactions to stress, fear and anxiety.
Money; asking, receiving, giving and withholding.
The elderly.
The sick; physically and mentally.
The fatherless family.
The unemployed man and his family.
Dishonest claimants.
The welfare functions of the Commission.
The structure of the social services: relations with social workers.

Some of this had already been taught in central training establishments; some had not. In any case the curriculum was replanned in order to integrate some of this material with technical and procedural instruction—a complex educational task. However there were two further areas that might help to develop and focus officers' skills, namely training in observation and an analysis of the discretionary aspects of the Executive Officers' work.

'Observation training' in the artificial situation of a central course can only be limited and must be related to training on the job. However it became apparent to the writer that the development of powers of observation was a matter of considerable importance in the overall programme. It is now well established that individuals vary greatly in the keenness of their observation, the elements they select and the inferences they draw from the observations.[1] The Supplementary Benefits official often needs to observe quickly and accurately in 'once and for all' situations. His work, especially that of the Clerical Officer, is so organised that he may only visit a particular claimant once but from his record of that visit a pattern may be set, by which subsequent observations by others may to an extent be determined. An officer's observations, for example, may start up a suspicion of abuse from which further investigations stem. The general condition of a house might suggest to one official that great efforts were being made to maintain a high standard of living on a small budget, to another that there were concealed resources. Similarly, the manner of a claimant might suggest to one an attempt to conceal the truth, to another anxiety leading to confusion about the facts. Thus 'observation training', which includes consideration of the subjective elements inherent in perception, may contribute to a more realistic appraisal of claimants and consequently to a weakening of the stereotyping based on clothing and appearance which officials often otherwise fall back on. Before the stage of inference is reached, it is necessary to encourage reliable and consistent observation. Central training courses now attempt to stimulate this by a variety of educational techniques, such as the use of closed circuit TV and videotape, but it is difficult to implement effectively at present.[2]

The general issue of the exercise of discretionary powers has been discussed at length in Chapter 2. There are three stages in a discretionary decision; first, the acquiring of information; second, making a judgement; and third, exercising a discretionary power. The first of these has occupied a central position in established training which a further emphasis on observation skills may complement. The second and third are at the root of much of the anxiety of new entrant Executive Officers but until recently have been considered only in relation to specific areas of the work, not in general terms as a principle of the Supplementary Benefits scheme and a most important element in practice. Central training course instructors now try to consider with their new entrants a number of general issues arising from their powers. In the field of exceptional needs grants, officials should be

[1] See, for example, M. L. J. Abercrombie *The Anatomy of Judgement: Investigation into the Processes of Perception and Reasoning*, Hutchinson, London, 1960; Penguin, Harmondsworth, 1969.

[2] It is understood that the present Social Work Adviser has plans for some experimental work in this medium.

helped to see how their own personal attitudes towards individual claimants, or towards particular categories of claimant, the differing material standards of an area, and the behaviour of the claimant, may play a part in the decision reached, as well as the objective facts of the need itself. The object of such discussion should be, of course, to increase objectivity through open acknowledgement of subjectivity. Underlying this is the assumption that a conscious and rational consideration of the difficulties involved in the exercise of discretion is desirable and that this is likely to be enhanced if training focuses attention on it in this way. Recent experience has shown that the new entrants have welcomed this emphasis. It may be that it will prove a more dynamic focus of concern for human relations teaching than the earlier 'dealing with people' sessions. The theme has now been introduced into courses for more senior officers.

Reference has been made earlier to the fact that these central courses are of a few weeks' duration only. The foregoing analysis of content demonstrates the difficulty of effective presentation of such material and discussion in the time available. The dangers of educational indigestion are obvious and the efficacy of a superficial introduction to these matters is unproven. Indeed, it may even be counter-productive if the presentation of such material is too restricted and it is somehow believed by those responsible for training to have been 'learnt' once and for all.

Furthermore, up until now this teaching has been carried out by the SBC instructors, highly skilled and knowledgeable in Supplementary Benefits administration, but not qualified in the teaching of many aspects of human relations. Very recently, attempts have been made at one centre to support the instructors through contact with the training staff of a local authority social services department. It is clearly a problem, however, how much working time such instructors can and should devote to the study of problems with which they themselves are not familiar, keeping abreast of new theory and trends in the social services as they come along. Without it, however, there is always a danger that human relations teaching will become rigid and outdated, contained within a structure which does not revitalise it. In short it would be fair to say that a sincere attempt has been made to incorporate into the central training of Supplementary Benefits officials those elements that are relevent to their attitudes towards claimants. Some of the serious difficulties in so doing are clear from the foregoing discussion. The role of the Social Work Adviser to the SBC is of considerable significance in such developments. Whatever the problems, however, it is of practical and symbolic significance that the SBC has acknowledged the importance of these aspects of training and is struggling to implement them within the framework of civil service training programmes; but such relatively limited schemes must not be allowed to mask some of the crucial and complex issues involved in achieving attitude change.

Impact of the Local Office on Staff Attitudes

New entrant Executive and Clerical Officers are usually assigned to area offices on first appointment. During the weeks preceding the central training course, they follow a training programme which is a combination of technical instruction, including programmed learning, visiting (accompanied and independent), and interviewing of callers. It is clear that this period is one which, if used constructively, might be significant in relation to the human relations aspect of training. It is likely to be a time of considerable emotional stress when the new recruit is receptive to fresh ideas. Indeed the influence of a local office may well be crucial in determining the new entrant's subsequent view of the job. His peers and his seniors—the people he turns to for advice and on whom his working contentment largely depends—are more important than instructors on central courses, however skilled. In the group dynamics and pressures of an office a few may stand out as non-conformers; but the majority will conform to what they believe to be the currently held values and norms. The 'reality shock' on the new recruit to Supplementary Benefits work must, of necessity, be considerable, especially on those who have led relatively sheltered lives. From the moment he arrives he will hear of every imaginable kind of human problem, distress and misconduct. Small wonder if he develops as quickly as possible a protective shell of cynicism to cope with this impact, especially is such cynicism is the generally accepted defence of the office. Therefore, this may be an opportunity for helping new entrants with the impact these experiences make upon him, to prevent the development of defences of a kind harmful to claimants.[1]

The period is also of crucial importance in the attempt to link theory, as presented on central courses, with practice as experienced in the local offices. This applies to all aspects of training, including procedural, but it is particularly important in those aspects of the work where formal attitudes and policies may appear to differ from or

---

[1] See and compare I. Mengies, 'The Functioning of Social Systems as a Defence against Anxiety', *Human Relations*, Vol. XIII. No. 2 (1960) for an analysis of the impact of painful situations upon nurses and hospitals and the defences that are adopted.

be in conflict with practice. In the small survey referred to previously, officers were asked to comment on the relationship between theory and practice. A very high percentage (about 80 per cent) of the Executive Officers believed that they could not carry out in practice what they had been taught on central courses. (Only about half the Clerical Officers thought so. This difference, once again, needs further study.) Among the comments from Executive Officers were the following:

'Theory can never foresee the variety of problems which can arise in welfare work. Different areas and towns have their different problems. Claimants are human and seldom conform to the codes as we do. Some rules and regulations are sensible in themselves but appear ridiculous to claimants as an explanation has to be taken out of context.'

'In theory we live in a utopia but in practice a large percentage of cases are potential frauds.'

'In theory a psychologist can work wonders on a man who is unemployed voluntarily. In practice, he is not mentally disturbed but realises that he is possibly better off financially when not working.'

'Theory cannot cover eventuality. It cannot fully take into account human reactions to certain situations nor always cover local problems.'

'Central Training often seems to forget there are unscrupulous people out to get every penny they can from the Ministry. It is difficult to consider a claimant's welfare when he is continually asking for grants etc. and refuses to make provision for these out of his allowance.'

'Theory does not teach the visiting officer to distinguish the genuine and not so genuine claimants and the course hardly touched on this. Practice teaches one that it needs a keen ear and eye and experience in the art of questioning to distinguish truth from fiction.'

Local Office Training Arrangements

Such comments raise fundamental educational issues concerned with the ways in which the Supplementary Benefits organisation seeks to influence the views and attitudes of officials. Neither instructions transmitted by codes nor instruction, however efficient, at central training courses, can be as potent a source of influence as the day-to-day local office regime. Yet, up till now, the approach to the development within local offices of the understanding of claimants, and skills in interviewing them, has been relatively unsophisticated. Practical experience has not been offered as a part of a systematic plan used as a basis for further training. This is partly due to the fragmentation of responsibility for training in local offices. At present, no one officer is designated to take particular responsibility for training. Overall responsibility for training his staff rests with the Manager who will delegate this in various ways. Executive Officers who are described as 'supervisors of clerical visiting' take the major responsibility for training the Clerical Officers who pay home visits and are sometimes in charge of the training programme in the tutelage period. Caller Executive Officers have taken less responsibility for the training of Clerical Officers. The Manager or Deputy expects to take some direct share in the training of Executive Officers through discussion and accompanied visiting but the new Executive Officer is normally assigned to a more experienced Executive Officer in the office, whom he is advised to consult on all points of difficulty. Instruction on various topics to both Executive and Clerical Officers and the supervision of programmed learning will be shared out between various Executive Officers and senior staff. These arrangements leave room for considerable variation between local offices. Managers vary greatly in the time and enthusiasm they devote to training and the ways in which they organise it internally. This is, of course, affected by, but not determined by, the pressure on any one office at particular points in time. There is, however, a vicious spiral in this, since a diminished investment in training can only lead to diminished efficiency and effectiveness, which in turn leads to further pressure or confusion. This applies as much to the areas of training with which this paper is concerned as to technical training.

Good managers show much concern for the welfare and training of their new staff. But as offices grow larger, as staff turnover increases, as the techniques of management become more complex and time-consuming, informal arrangements are not adequate to meet the training needs. Managers spoke to the writer of telling new Executive Officers that 'their door was always open'. But what if the new Executive Officer is too nervous to poke his head round or the Manager seems to be for ever on the telephone? Similarly, the informal arrangements made with the experienced Executive Officer is full of hazards. If he is harassed, will a new Executive Officer feel able to bother his senior? What if, in a particular office, the most experienced Executive Officer has been in post for a very short time? The 'brother' Executive

Officer has no formal allowance of time for his training responsibility, which is bound to affect his attitude to the task and that of the trainee. Furthermore the fact that the two officers are of equal grade, although there will normally be differences in age and seniority, is an unusual situation is a service in which authority and grade are closely linked. It seems, therefore, that some greater degree of formality in the arrangements made for the training of Executive Officers is essential.

The position with regard to Clerical Officer training is structurally less confused in that the role of the Executive Officers concerned is defined and their responsibility for training accepted. The structure requires a Clerical Officer to work to an Executive Officer whereas the Executive Officer has considerable independence. In this way, the training relationship is affected.

New Models for Local Office Training

The differences between the size of local office, their particular conditions, the interest of Managers in training, and the calibre of staff available for training, all make for difficulties in laying down formal patterns which would be appropriate for all and there is an understandable reluctance to encroach too far on Managers' independence. The notion of a 'training officer' in each local office is not favoured since it is believed that it would undermine a fundamental principle of a combined responsibility for supervision and training among various members of staff. The fact remains that the present situation has one most unfortunate consequence—the good reinforces the good, the bad reinforces the bad. The appointment in the near future of Social Work Service Officers in the s b c is likely to have a significant effect on some aspects of local office training and may help to establish continuity in teaching about human relations. Even so, from an organisational point of view, it would seem that to ensure reasonable consistency, recent developments in training units independent of local offices are likely to be necessary in improving standards. However, any such arrangements or changes in the internal organisation of local offices leaves unaltered the basic educational problem—how best to socialise the official at field level into the role the s b c wishes him to acquire. Limited as the objectives may be in comparison with those for the professional, such training is intended, as with social workers, to increase knowledge and skill and to modify attitudes. So far as skill and attitudes are concerned, educational techniques must be devised that take account of the learning processes of individuals, their varying reactions to and defences against the situations and claimants they meet. In short, training that seeks to individualise the needs and problems of claimants must also individualise the needs and problems of the officials, insofar as these are relevant to the task he is being asked to perform. Otherwise it is a contradiction in terms and may even serve to increase cynicism and distrust of official policy regarding welfare.

In many ways, such a notion is incompatible with a traditional bureaucratic system in which obedience to authority has tended to inhibit challenge, even discussion, and in which local office training has been based on a model of apprenticeship. That is to say, it has been assumed that there is a reasonably clear distinction between right and wrong modes of behaviour and that such distinctions can be imparted by 'a watch and follow technique'. Thus, for example, interviewing is learnt by 'accompanied visits' in which first tutor, then pupil, demonstrate their skills. It seems that in training, as in so many aspects of the Supplementary Benefits scheme, the administration is attempting, somewhat uneasily, to combine a bureaucratic and a professional style. The task to be performed does not require full professional expertise, since the degree of individual initiative and responsibility is not so great. Yet the knowledge, skills and attitudes required are similar and lead to consideration of educational techniques similar to those now employed by the helping professions. If there are to be sensitivity groups for social workers, psychiatrists, GPs and nurses—and indeed for many branches of industrial management—why not for Supplementary Benefits officials? To pose the question is not to advocate that particular technique. The improbability of such an experiment at present does, however, serve to emphasise the gulf that still exists, despite much conscientious effort, between the conception of training as perceived by the Supplementary Benefits official and, for example, social workers. Essentially this is a dichotomy between a view of the trainee as a 'rational man' who will be persuaded by rational instruction and a view of him as in part irrational, needing to be persuaded by techniques which take account of his irrational and unconscious feelings and which encourage expression of feeling as a means to that end. This matters more for some branches of the civil servants' work than for others. (Indeed, for some it might be a positive hindrance to the work.) In fields such as supplementary benefits, however, training for attitude change, which is crucial to the use of knowledge and the development of skill, should be planned and evaluated in the context of similar training elsewhere. Of course training methods come in and go out of favour and there is much that is uncertain and frankly dubious in this field at present. It would seem, however, that for human rela-

N

tions to take an effective place in the total Supplementary Benefits training programme, there must be an acceptance of the powerful forces working against such an orientation. These are in part the product of the individual's own particular attitudes, compounded of fear, anxiety, antagonism and envy of some claimants; in part they are generated by group feelings and, on occasion, by the fear of alienation from the group.

Such considerations might lead to a variety of experiments in local office training, of which the most obvious is a form of supervision similar, although not identical, to that which has been developed in social work. The fears among social work students and some staff that this will involve unwarrantable intrusion into their private feelings is one which would probably be experienced even more intensely by Supplementaty Benefits officials, who are totally unaccustomed to such procedures. Although British social work has avoided the worst excesses of pseudo psycho-analytic techniques in its supervision, the fears have some foundation in reality in that once the principle is established that 'work behaviour' is related to personal feelings and individuals, it follows that in a sense 'intrusion' is inevitable, even if it is firmly focused upon the job that has to be done. Against that must be placed the relief experienced by many in talking about their interaction with those they are trying to help. There is no reason to suppose that Supplementary Benefits officials would be any exception, although the question of sanctions for such a form of training needs to be considered. It is true that intending social workers do not 'sanction' such aspects of their education. But they usually have a role expectation which would lead them to accept the importance of the supervisory process. This is not the case with the Supplementary Benefits trainee whose perception of the task he will be undertaking may not include consideration of the human relations aspect; in any case he may not have chosen to do this work.

A further difficulty in adapting a model based upon social work supervision for Supplementary Benefits officials lies in the authoritive connotation of this term for them and the expectations of a relationship with authority. This in turn raises the question as to who should provide the supervision. To avoid inappropriate extrapolation from social work, it would be desirable to use officials. It remains to be seen, however, if supervisory techniques of this kind can be acquired by those to whom they are strange and which are in some ways antipathetic to the accepted normative behaviour of those in authority.

Reference to this particular educational method is intended to illustrate possibilities that the sbc might explore in relation to training in local offices. It is not intended to imply that a model of social work supervision is a panacea. Within social work, supervision needs to be developed, modified and above all evaluated. Its application to the supplementary benefits field is even more uncertain and can only be discovered by experiment—which was suggested to the sbc by the writer. What seems absolutely certain, however, is that rational man, rationally instructed, will not alone suffice. This form of supervision offers a possibility of integration of formal policies with day-to-day practice.[1]

So far as relations with the social services are concerned, local office training could have much to contribute. Managers are encouraged to arrange staff meetings for specific purposes, including invitations to representatives of outside organisations, such as social workers. However, it was the writer's impression that this was rare. Such meetings, together with visits by officers to other departments and agencies seem an important part of training, to avoid 'in-breeding'. Recently one local authority social service department has offered short observational placements to Supplementary Benefits officers in training. The advantages of expanding this need no argument.

To improve local office training poses the Supplementary Benefits administrators with complex problems of organisation far more difficult to resolve than those created by changes in central courses. Furthermore, they take one into more subtle, less tangible matters in which it is harder to define objectives and assess results. Those responsible for training have less control than they have over central or regional courses. The authority of the Manager must not be undermined; the organisation of training has to be seen in relation to office organisation as a whole; and offices will vary, according to personnel, at different points in time and between themselves, in their attitudes to 'human relations' training. It is not, therefore, surprising that progress in these matters has been comparatively slow. But it is at the core of the enterprise.

Regional Training

At present regional centres provide a variety of short technical specialist courses according to local needs. They also provide refresher and remedial courses. The development of regional training since 1966 has

---

[1] This is to be further explored by the Social Work Adviser and the Social Work Service Officers.

been a significant factor. Before the integration of the NAB and MPNI, there was no regional training provided by the NAB. In 1970 the regional courses for SBC staff amounted to 17,545 days. Examples of topics included: assessment, counter interviewing, visiting, liable relative work, appeals, and fraud, in addition to the refresher courses referred to earlier. Clearly, much of what has been said in relation to the two central courses will apply equally to regional centres that are confronted with the same problems. In some ways, however, their task is harder since they have a smaller number of experienced instructors suitable to cover 'human relations' training and have been more closely identified with the National Insurance aspects of social security. However, the need for 'human relations' training has become apparent to most in the five years since the merger. Within some regions there are particular social problems that have a direct bearing on supplementary benefits work: for example, the presence of immigrant communities or the drift to certain areas of young, unattached people. Sometimes there will be associated technical problems: for example, in determining cohabitation in the case of West Indian women, for which understanding of the cultural factors may be of practical help and of importance in reducing prejudice[1] or in exercising discretion in relation to the 'drifters' who claim benefit. Regional centres may have a part to play in such aspects of human relations training not least because of the economy of time which such localised training affords. Regional training might also be expected to play a part in experiments in local office training. It is important not to underemphasise the role of regional centres in a training programme. Regional offices act as a filter between local offices and 'Headquarters' and, apart from the central training courses, officials at field level communicate upwards via regional offices on all matters. Thus the significance of attitudes within regional offices towards supplementary benefits work is considerable and this, in turn, is reflected in training. This is one of the reasons why the appointment of Regional Social Work Service Officers is important.

Specialised Training

There are four specialisms of particular concern in the context of this discussion; Special Welfare Officers, Unemployment Review Officers, Liable Relative Officers and Managers of Reception and or Re-establishment Centres.

[1] A booklet has now been issued to officials about the cultural problems of immigrants.

Special Welfare Officers

Special Welfare Officers have, since they were first appointed, attended short courses arranged at Headquarters. However, it is only since 1969 that such courses have been developed in cooperation with outside educational establishments and tutored by social work teachers.[1] As was argued earlier,[2] the role of the swo is virtually indistinguishable from that of a social worker and it is, therefore, desirable that their training should be in the hands of social work educators. However, as more social workers become trained, the inadequacy of the short courses offered to the swos will become more obvious and this will call in question the whole basis of the specialism. Although the Commission have accepted in principle the social work role of the swos, the full implications of this for training have not yet been acknowledged. This is partly, as was discussed earlier, because swos will not remain within this specialism indefinitely and there is a fear that a long training would be wasted. Behind this, one suspects, lurks a continuing doubt as to the need for and value of such education. It may well be, therefore, that the issue of training will eventually force into the open the inconsistency of a policy which establishes roles without the professional structure within which swos should operate. Similar developments to those for swos are beginning for the staff of Re-establishment and Reception Centres. During 1971 the tutors of the social work department of a polytechnic organised and ran three fortnight residential courses for them.

Unemployment Review Officers

Unemployment Review Officers did not, until recently, receive specialised training. Here again, however, short courses which all uros attend are now arranged in cooperation with a university department of social work. To those accustomed to such arrangements, these developments will not seem spectacular, especially in view of the short periods of time available to convey complex and wide-ranging information and understanding. Their importance, however, is considerable in establishing a principle that the sbc will seek outside professional assistance from independent educational institutions. The

---

[1] These are now moving into another phase as a two-part course. Part 1, a non-residential fortnight based at the London Training Headquarters is organised and run by the Social Work Adviser; Part II, which follows a few months later, is a residential fortnight organised and run by a university social work department. Further links and continuity will be provided by the Social Work Service Officers.

[2] See chapter 7.

most significant gain is the move from the 'closed' to the 'open' system. This could have effects that go far beyond the actual impact of such education on individual officers. Their very existence means that a relationship is created between officials responsible for training and their senior administrators and the academics, especially those who teach social work. The ignorance of each about the other must be a matter of concern and, in a small way, these courses can contribute to mutual understanding. On the other hand, it is possible that they will play a part in creating more open conflict both within the SBC and between the SBC and social workers. For 'the specialists'—SWos and UROs—may, as a result of interaction with social work educators and social scientists, become more aware of role confusion and role conflict, as discussed in earlier chapters. This may be a healthy stimulus to clarification or even to a change in roles but it is doubtful whether this side-effect has been anticipated and much will depend on the response of the hierarchy to challenge. So far as relations with social workers are concerned, greater knowledge of the workings of the Supplementary Benefits scheme may promote more informed criticism than has hitherto been evident. If responsibility is given to outsiders to run courses they must be given information to help them to do so. Therefore among a small but potentially influential group there will be knowledge which, while not secret, has not been made available before.

Liable Relative Officers

Most Liable Relative Officers receive specialised training but it is of a technical nature. (There is a considerable amount of legal technical information that must be acquired.) As has already been indicated, the LRO has not, until recently, been encouraged through training, to consider in any depth the implications of his task for the welfare of claimants. However, this is now under review and it seems probable that there will be changes in length and content that will enable more time to be devoted to human relations.

University Courses in Human Relations and the Social Services

Reference was made at the beginning of this chapter to the place of these courses in an overall programme of staff development and to the fact that considerable numbers of officers have, in the past fifteen to twenty years, attended them.

A starting point in thinking about such courses should be the part they play, or should play, in the total educational programme for the Commission's officers. At present, it is the writer's impression that there is some confusion and ambiguity about this, which leads to uncertainty about the degree of relevance they have—or ought to have—to the day-to-day work. Such ambiguity may lead to disappointment for both the teacher and the taught. The issue is further complicated by the terms of reference of extra-mural departments, which organise many of the courses and have a specifically non-vocational charter from the Department of Education and Science which enables them to claim grant aid. (There are, however, considerable differences in how rigidly this is interpreted.) Thus, ultimately, one may view these courses as of broad educational value but essentially as no different from evening classes in any other subject, from music to politics; or one may strive for a narrow definition of relevance in which the subjects rest fairly and squarely on the direct concerns of the Supplementary Benefits officer. Both these views are extreme. The courses can and should provide knowledge and understanding, which is of use to the work, but in essence that they should not seek to imitate inservice training and to provide what should properly be included within the normal training structure of the SBC. The remarks of some officials to the writer suggested that they were disappointed with some of the courses on the grounds that they were of insufficient relevance to the task. One heard of the difference between courses that were 'too academic' and those in which tutors 'have their feet on the ground'. This may mean that the teaching is pitched at too high or too abstruse a level—in which case it is clearly an educational weakness; or it may mean that narrow focus has been expected because central and regional training has not had the time and resources to do its own job effectively. It is clear, however, that these courses should be planned in the context of decisions regarding central and regional training and in relation to those elements that are to be regarded as essential to the inservice programme.

There are a number of detailed issues involved in the success or failure of these classes which it is beyond the scope of this chapter to consider. These include: the composition and location of the classes; the qualifications of the teachers; curriculum planning; and the length and pattern of courses. Such details raise, however, more fundamental questions as to the relationship that exists between those who initiate, plan, and teach on the courses. There are often, although not always, three parties involved in the organisation of such courses: the Department of Social Security; the extra-mural department of a university or the WEA, the university department, usually of social studies, in which the tutors work. This may on occasion complicate communications between the Department of Health and Social Security and the tutors.

The responsibility within the Department of Health and Social Security for initiating courses rests with the Regional Training Officer, who is concerned with all aspects of social security training. Most RTOs have come from the National Insurance side of the Department and SBC training occupies a smaller part of their time, of which extra-mural courses are a minute part.

Most RTOs would be the first to admit that they are a little uneasy about their position. They have not the professional knowledge enabling them to discuss content and planning in any great depth and they have many other demands on their time. Inevitably, the courses tend to be seen as peripheral to their main concerns. In short, the problem as in so many other matters, lies in the uneasiness in relations between the administrator and the professional. This will probably be improved by the introduction of 'a professional element' into the SBC and may be an important part of the new Regional Social Work Officer's task.

To conclude; the present pattern of training—central, local, regional and specialist has been described; the case for 'human relations' training at all levels has been argued, but the difficulties of ensuring that it is meaningful and effective are considerable in an organisation of this kind which is unaccustomed to using such knowledge. To be successful, such training must be clearly focused upon the task but must also be set within the context of wider programmes of staff development.

CHAPTER 9

RELATIONS WITH SOCIAL WORKERS—
PRESENT AND FUTURE

In a sense the whole of this book has been concerned with relations between the s b c and social work. The preceding chapters have attempted to analyse the basic issues involved in the separation of income maintenance services from social work. The assumption on which separation of services is based is that it is desirable to keep an individual's financial need and entitlement apart from his social and psychological need and entitlement. It has been shown that the arguments in favour of this are powerful and the dangers of any system that confuses the two very considerable. Nonetheless there is abundant evidence that the separation creates a multiplicity of difficulties for the minority of claimants for whom these needs are interwined. This minority are those with whom social work is, or should be, concerned. They would exist whatever structure of social service were created. The questions one must consider are; whether our present structure is, in general and in theory, as good or better than any other we might devise; whether the theory is reasonably congruent with the practice; and what further improvements may be made to the existing structures. This chapter will discuss in some detail matters arising from these fundamental questions but, before doing so, the attitudes of social workers to the s b c will be considered and related to trends in social work at the present time.

Confrontation

The 'poverty lobby' in social work, on which the Child Poverty Action Group has been an important influence, is a predictable and useful reaction to excessive preoccupation with psychological factors in social difficulty. It is one of the elements that has recently served to redress the balance in social casework. However these developments have more far-reaching repercussions since they lead to an awareness of defects in the social structure as such, for which social casework may seem inappropriate or even harmful. They contribute, therefore, to movements for community or political action and to the organisation of pressure groups. There are signs that this is resulting in a more articulate and militant strategy amongst some social workers in their relationship to government, be it local or central. The dilemmas this poses for the professional within a bureaucracy are well known and much discussed.

As part of this trend it seems inevitable that there will be a greater degree of confrontation between social work as a profession and the SBC, just as there will be between the professions and local government. The probable effects of this are hard to gauge and much depends on the issues chosen for confrontation and the manner in which this is staged. There is no doubt that any organisation tends to protect the status quo and to be resistant to change. Government bureaucracies show this tendency to a marked degree and the SBC is not immune. Thus there may well be issues for which organised pressure of this kind brings the only hope of change. At the same time it would be totally wrong to suppose that the SBC and its administrators are insensitive to criticism unless it is dramatically and publicly proclaimed. On the contrary, the most detailed and searching examination is made of individual cases and of specific policy issues when criticisms are received. The concern of the higher civil servant in the SBC to see that justice—as he sees it—has been done is beyond reproach. The difficulty lies in the gap that may exist between official policy and local office practice. We enter here into the realm of subjective impressions, of reports of the handling of particular cases in which facts are only part of the story and in which the perceptions of claimants, social workers, and officials may be at variance. Senior officials may on occasion receive one-sided accounts of events and there is a natural tendency to defend their own colleagues. The traditional reporting of civil servants, with its emphasis on 'hard facts' to the exclusion of 'soft facts', does not facilitate understanding of the total situation.

There are basic issues of policy on which confrontation is both proper and appropriate. It is, however, the impression of the writer that many of the most disturbing areas of conflict between the SBC and social workers lie, not in the realms of official policy, but in the ways policy is believed by social workers to be implemented—or not implemented. In such situations it is difficult to achieve results by a strategy of confrontation: first, because the evidence available is usually confused and open to different interpretations; secondly, because there tends to be a hardening of attitudes on both sides when criticisms of individuals are involved. (Social workers might be expected to understand that behaviour is rarely modified by attack.) Thirdly, where the real issue is the policy itself rather than the local offices' interpretation of it, confrontation at local level may be quite inappropriate. Thus it seems important to distinguish these issues for which the confrontation technique is appropriate and those for which it is counterproductive. This is no simple matter, however. For if social workers believe that the gap between policy and practice is intolerable and that the policy is impossible to implement with due regard to welfare, then they must attack practice to make their point. It then becomes important to ensure that such criticism is based on a proper understanding of the law and regulations behind the operations of the SBC and on a realistic appraisal of the evidence of particular cases. Otherwise, regrettably but understandably, officials tend to become sceptical and resentful of the protests. There is considerable evidence that social workers tend to be inaccurate and vague in their allegations.

'Openness' in Government

Probably the most healthy aspect of relations between social work and the SBC lies in the increasing openness of the latter to discuss and disclose matters of policy. There are different reasons for this. It may be a part of a general trend in government, a welcome increase in concern for democratic debate. Pressures such as those by the Child Poverty Action Group may also have been significant. It may be that the introduction of a social work element into the SBC has played its part. The influence of Commission members themselves should not be underestimated; they may be counted as among the more progressive and concerned members of the establishment. Certainly, the publication of the Supplementary Benefits Handbook, the papers on the wage stop and cohabitation and others which are forthcoming can do much to make the debate between the two a more informed one than has hitherto been the case. For one of the most unfortunate aspects of relations between Supplementary Benefits and social work has been the sheer ignorance of the frames of reference, governed by statute, the regulations, roles, training and ultimately the value systems, each of the other. In this an older generation of social workers, orientated towards the psychological rather than towards the practical, have been more at fault than new-style radicals, for they have grumbled without pinpointing with accuracy the source of their discontent and without organised protest. The activists, on the other hand, have awakened interest in the details of Supplementary Benefits policy and performance, in a dimension of their clients' wellbeing which is of critical importance. The real danger, nonetheless, lies in the need of both elements in social work *not* to understand some of the subtleties of policy and the intricacies of procedure, lest *tout comprendre, c'est tout pardonner*. Social action does not thrive on understanding the point of view of authority and the potency of social work may in some situations have been reduced by conciliatory attitudes. Some of the criticism of the Supplementary Benefits scheme and, in particular, of officials' attitudes, takes less account of the difficulties—some of which have been discussed in this book—that might be expected of social workers whom one would imagine would not usually resort to such over-simplications. Could it be that social workers, compelled to be tolerant of so much and so many, find in the sbc a convenient scapegoat? To preserve a scapegoat, it is essential not to understand.

Thus it comes about that the social workers' need not to understand has interacted unhealthily with the sbc's bureaucratic reticence. This has been fostered by a total structural division not only between social workers and officials but between units of government—local and central. Furthermore, these units of government do not even coincide with one another geographically and, until the creation of the social service departments, the Supplementary Benefits official has been required to deal, not only with different local authorities, but with several social work departments within these local authorities in addition to other branches of the social services such as housing or education. The variation in policy and procedure between and within local authorities needs no elaboration here. Its effect on cooperation and on the attitudes of Supplementary Benefits staff to social workers has been considerable. When one adds to this the differences of emphasis between individualised and equitable justice, one can see that by the creation of the National Assistance Board in 1948, the stage was set for confusion, misunderstanding and conflict. The celebrations that greeted its birth now have a hollow ring. However, in recent years, it has become clear that those in higher authority on both sides have a growing appreciation of the difficulties and of their importance. There is evidence of efforts by the sbc to improve relations and a greater degree of communication about areas of difficulty. That this is bearing fruit may be indicated by a recent survey undertaken by the former Children's Officers Association which, although critical, suggested an improvement in comparison with the findings of a similar study undertaken five years ago.[1]

---

[1] Private communication to the sbc.

Ministerial Amalgamation

It is possible also that the arbitrary, politically-inspired, merger of the Ministry of Social Security and the Ministry of Health will have some surprising beneficial side-effects. For this was followed in 1971 by the unification of central government responsibility for social services (excluding the probation service) in the same department as the Supplementary Benefits administration. Despite the complexities of this large and unwieldy structure and of the inevitable reorganisation attendant upon mergers and transfers, it is likely that the social workers in central government will now become more aware of, and involved in, relations with the SBC and that this will promote better cooperation at local government level. In this connection, it should be noted that the permanent Social Work Adviser to the SBC is now a member of the social work service of the Department of Health and Social Security. The post is the only one directly involved with social work matters in this central government department; all the others are concerned with the links with local government. Part of the Supplementary Benefit Social Work Officer's task is to increase knowledge of the SBC's work *within* the central government social work service. Currently, appointments are being made of social work service officers who will work under the professional direction of the Social Work Adviser but will operate within the regional structure.

Defensive Posture of Civil Servants

Perhaps it is in the nature of things that, although Supplementary Benefits baiting has become a favourite pastime of some social workers, the bear has not been able to retaliate. It is a curious one-sided situation which derives in part from the traditions of the British civil service.[1] More often than not 'improvements in relations' means to social workers improvements in administration or policy concessions on the part of the SBC. The civil servants for the most part are on the defensive. True to their name, they seek to serve with varying degrees of formal and informal responsiveness but rarely, if ever, indulge in open criticism of those to whom they are required to relate. Yet, as everyone knows, social work is a very long way from providing the services needed to complement material and financial assistance. One wonders whether the attacking and defensive postures of social work and the SBC respectively are the best way of achieving better understanding.

[1] By contrast, for example, some Israeli civil servants write freely to the press in their own name criticising what they will.

Field Level Communications

Whatever useful communications may develop at the higher levels on both sides, it is at the field level that success of communication must ultimately be judged. During 1968 and 1969, in the inquiries made of five professional Associations,[1] an assessment of this was made. Furthermore, social services in three county boroughs, widely separated geographically, were studied by the writer. To these impressions have been added many personal communications of various kinds and, more recently, the views of Children's Officers. The following assessment, therefore, of relations existing between 1968 and the present time is not derived solely from an articulate minority, important as their views may be.

Social Workers' Knowledge of the Supplementary Benefits scheme

The professional associations were asked a number of questions and it is upon these that the following discussion is based, although the comments are not solely derived from the associations.

Are the statutory powers, limits and allowances adequately understood by social workers?

The short, unequivocal answer to this question is 'No'—an answer given by nearly all of the associations consulted and amply borne out by interviews with social workers and by evidence from other sources. Some of the responsibility rests, as has been suggested earlier, with the bias (until recently) of the profession and the deficiencies of social work education in this field. However this is not the whole story as the Commission recognised in the decision to publish a handbook primarily for social workers. The feeling has been, as one association put it, that the Commission has 'tended to shroud its affairs in mystery' and this impression may have been strengthened by the tendency of inexperienced and unsure officers in local offices to 'play it close to the chest' in case they should be wrong. It seems therefore that improvements in social workers' knowledge of the scheme are an essential preliminary to any other improvements in relationships of a more subtle kind.

Communications Between Officials and Social Workers

Are the communications between SBC officials and social workers adequate to ensure: (a) reasonably good general relationships, (b) clarification and/or solution of conflict over individual cases?

A number of different ingredients go into the establishment of success-

[1] See chapter 2.

ful communications in which a problem is clarified or solved. Among these ingredients are: first, accessibility; secondly, mutual respect and understanding of the other's role; thirdly, shared concern for the object of the exercise, the client/claimant; fourthly, some degree of flexibility. These four elements are, of course, inextricably involved with each other. However the last three are more complex aspects of communication considered under the headings of other questions in this chapter and have been explored to some extent in earlier chapters. The issue of accessibility, however, is at least in part a practical and organisational one and it is therefore of interest to consider the ways in which local offices organise contact and communication with social workers and vice versa.

Practical matters, trivial in themselves, contribute to the success or failure of communications. Thus, for example, the handling of incoming telephone calls may affect the confidence each feels in the other. Social workers on occasion speak to Clerical Assistants or Clerical Officers and sometimes subsequently find the details of the case have not been fully understood or a helpful answer given. In such cases the Clerical Officer is not empowered to take decisions and may well know nothing of the case.[1] A number of social workers expressed reluctance to call at the office because of the lack of privacy for conversations. It was clear from the opinions expressed by social workers that local Supplementary Benefits offices varied considerably in the arrangements they made for dealing with social workers' inquiries, although this is said to have improved since the study was undertaken.

However, behind such practical considerations (which are nonetheless extremely important in increasing or decreasing tensions), there are more fundamental problems of communication. Reference has already been made to the bewildering complexity of the services with which the Supplementary Benefits official has had in the past to deal—still only simplified to a limited extent. There is also a difficulty for him in direct personal contact with social workers. Executive Officers, of course, vary in levels of ability: but the position is much more confusing in relation to social workers. It is possible for an Executive Officer to be speaking one moment to a graduate of high ability with full professional qualifications and the next moment to a worker with no formal educational qualifications whatsoever and no training—and all other permutations and combinations, including unintelligent, untrained graduates! Similarly, some doubts exist in the minds of social

[1] See Chapter 3.

workers as to the appropriate level of communication with local offices. In short, the question arises—who is my opposite number? There is not a straightforward answer to this. Social work departments are organised with varying degrees of professional autonomy according to their structure; thus, a Probation Officer expects to take almost total responsibility for his case, a local authority social worker works within a more defined hierarchy. Both, however, are expected—and expect—to have a greater degree of autonomy in many respects than the Clerical or Executive Officer, within a more formal bureaucratic structure. This can lead to mutual irritation and misunderstanding. It also leads to sympathetic social workers being worried about 'going above the officer's head' when disagreeing with a decision. Thus there may be reluctance to go to the Manager or Deputy over a dispute with an Executive Officer. This is bound to make for insecurity in the approaches each makes to the other. It may be that some social workers are unnecessarily sensitive with regard to consulting higher levels in the organisation; for although there will be some human resentment, the notion of upward referral in cases of disagreement is well established in government bureaucracy. There is certainly strong reluctance in social workers to approach regional offices direct, it being felt that this would prejudice local relationships. (It should also be noted in passing, however, that many social workers were unaware of the regional structure anyway). The use of the Appeals Tribunal is often seen as the next, and only, logical step when a local office, in the opinion of the social worker, does not give satisfaction and the possibility of further discussion with regional offices is rarely considered. It seems that, without undermining the authority and autonomy of the local office manager, the channels of communication about policy matters between senior officials in social work departments and the regional staff could in some areas be opened up further to mutual advantage; this is being actively encouraged by Headquarters.

Welfare Referral

An important aspect of communication concerns welfare referral. The Supplementary Benefits officer has a duty to advise the claimant of the appropriate social service agency in those cases in which the need becomes apparent in the course of his financial investigation. (Where the claimant is not capable of acting on advice, the official is instructed to get in touch with the agency himself.) Much of this book has been concerned with complex and problematical aspects of people in social difficulty. However there are many cases in which the welfare need is relatively straightforward and, especially in the case of elderly people, involves no controversy between the official and the social worker. At present, this referral is usually done by telephone but the frustrations of telephone communication are well known. It is possible that, for simple referrals that are not urgent, a written referral might be preferable—possibly some simple proforma agreed with the local agencies. The suggestion is not as trivial as it sounds. Such an arrangement would have two main advantages: first, it would increase the reliability of referral, for such a device would surely be no more time-consuming than phone calls; secondly, it would help to ensure that the information supplied on referral was what the agency needed, thus in effect educating the official in the task of referral. It would also be desirable for the social worker to convey, however briefly, the outcome of the referral. (Supplementary Benefits officials commented that they scarcely ever knew what action followed their referral.) This feedback is crucially important if the policy of welfare referral is to be implemented in practice, for officials cannot maintain interest in a vacuum. Once again this communication is more likely to take place if it is formalised (as simply as possible) and it may afford an opportunity of pointing out unsuitable referrals. For example, it was apparent from inquiries that Supplementary Benefits officials on occasion felt angry that so little (apparently) was done for the mentally ill whom they had referred. It is possible that this was sometimes due to an exaggerated hope of what could be done in such cases. Finally, some formal system of referral, which is difficult in the present hit-and-miss arrangements, would also lend itself to evaluation and discussion of local arrangements.

Behind these simple practical points lies the obvious but neglected fact that, the separation having been created, the problems of communication that arise have to be worked at—especially as the respective organisations become more complex and most particularly in dense urban areas which throw up the greatest number of social problems and in which the numbers and turnover of staff on both sides are greater. Effective referral in straightforward cases contributes more than alleviation of the need of a particular individual: it engenders confidence and trust which can then be drawn upon when difficulties arise.

Communication, however, is affected by the values and attitudes of the parties as well as by organisation. Thus, a further question was put to the Associations.

Particular Difficulties with Certain Claimants

Are there some types of client or problem over which difficulties arise between social workers and SBC officials and to what do you attribute these difficulties?

As one might expect, the summary of the replies given by the professional associations indicated concern about the way in which those whom we might describe as 'the undesirables' are treated, whether they be problem families, alcoholics, vagrants, unmarried mothers or any of those whose behaviour may give rise to moral outrage. One association summed it up thus: 'The types of client over which difficulties commonly arise are those where problems arise because of emotional factors which are difficult to accept and understand without specialised knowledge'. No useful purpose is served by attempting to gloss over the indications of prejudice against certain individuals or 'types' and the justice of the social workers' criticisms in a number of instances. However, these are intangible areas and therefore more difficult, if not impossible, to prove. One of the difficulties is that the social workers sometimes depend on the reports of clients among whom there are dishonest and difficult people, sometimes adept at playing officials off one against the other. Some social workers are fully aware of this and take it into account when making criticisms; others are more gullible. However, whatever the justice of the criticism in general, it is a widely held view and widely talked about by social workers—that there are sorts of people who get 'a raw deal' from Supplementary Benefits. How much this affects the money they actually receive is, of course, another issue. But if the feeling exists among the section of the social services with which the Supplementary Benefits Commission has to work most closely that prejudice does exist, it warrants, first, careful study of its extent and an attempt to correct it where it exists and secondly, a programme to improve the image of the Supplementary Benefits officer in the eyes of the social workers. As has been shown, there are real difficulties over differences of role and function which arise over issues such as cohabitation and voluntary unemployment. But all the difficulties cannot be attributed to valid differences of approach. The attitude that some officials do adopt, the distinction between 'deserving and undeserving', the distaste, even disgust that may be felt at certain types of person or problem—all these are perfectly normal 'lay' reactions to the impact of this work. The traditional impartiality of the bureaucrat who may be relied upon to make objective decisions in the light of available evidence, carefully weighted and sifted, is simply not adequate to cope with the decisions that must be taken in a variety of complex and sometimes sordid situations; anxiety about abuse may act as a further irritant in an already difficult face-to-face situation. (It is of interest to note that the social workers particularly criticised 'counter staff' in answering this question.)

However, there may have to be certain broad differences of emphasis between Supplementary Benefits officials and social workers in the degree of concern for 'protecting the public purse' or 'the welfare of the underdog'. Each side can point to a different kind of naivety in the other. As one Executive Officer put it: 'Social workers are airy-fairy. They have faith in everybody, whereas Supplementary Benefits officers have faith in nobody'. Over-simplified and crude as this may be, it highlights a real situation. There were some social workers who, in addition to being ignorant of their claimant's financial affairs, were extraordinarily naive in accepting what claimants told them without verification. For example, one complaint from a Children's Department concerned the refusal of Supplementary Benefits to pay storage charges on furniture. This, it was suggested, forced the claimant to work in the evenings when she should have been looking after her infant son. Examination of the case paper showed that these charges had been met from the beginning. It is possible that the claimant told the social worker she had to work in the evenings and gave this as an excuse. There were other cases where it was at least possible that the social workers were withholding knowledge of additional sources of income from the local offices. This kind of situation poses a complex ethical problem. The social worker is bound to respect the confidences of his client, as any other professional, and there could be no question of automatically 'swopping' information with Supplementary Benefits— nor would Supplementary Benefits officers divulge certain information either. However the situation is not as simple as that. Is there a moral obligation on the social worker to encourage his client to disclose alternative sources of income to officials? This is not always felt to be an obligation: the encouragement may be merely lip service. This, on occasions, springs from a total identification with 'the underdog' against established authority and it is arguable that this is to the detriment of the client. But Supplementary Benefits officials must also, in some instances, take their share of blame. For if the image of a particular local office is Scrooge-like, if the witholding of money is felt by the social workers to be the dominant emphasis, then it is easy to see that the fight on behalf of clients can come to include an acceptance that they must get what they can from whatever source without too many questions being asked. The ignorance of social workers about the Supplementary Benefits scheme, however, undoubtedly contributes to the problem. For in some instances a proper and reasonable application of the regulations—as, for example, in some wage stop cases—raises the ire of social workers against local offices when it should properly be directed elsewhere, at the wages structure of low-paid workers, for example. In other cases, their feelings that local offices are mean may be justified. But Supplementary Benefits officials are sometimes in possession of knowledge which they cannot divulge to social workers, which would explain what is felt by the social workers to be 'meanness'—undisclosed earnings being an obvious example. Then, when the social workers protest, they are accused of being naive. Yet the officials may equally, on occasion, be called naive for over-simplifying, for example, a complex marital situation and suspecting fictitious desertion when all the social and psychological circumstances point to the contrary. We can all point to instances which contradict the Executive Officer's remark that the social workers have faith in everybody whereas Supplementary Benefits officers have faith in nobody. Put in general terms, however, the observation is worth taking seriously, arising as it does from a complex interaction of motivation for different kinds of work, training, and perhaps most important of all, the orientation and frame of reference of the job.

Procedural Difficulties
Do difficulties arise over procedural matters which in your opinion affect clients' welfare?
The evidence is strong that there is fairly widespread concern among social workers on this point: reference is made to delays in visiting, long waiting periods in offices, difficulty over emergency payments and so on. It seems to the writer that this is one of the issues on which organised pressure and protest can be most effective. Criticism of this kind can be backed by concrete evidence: it attacks the cherished values of the civil servant for whom reliability and efficiency are the primary virtues and, as such, receives meticulous attention; and it can be improved by technical and procedural changes about which the senior officials of the SBC are much concerned. Perhaps most important of all, informed criticism of this kind lends weight to arguments for much needed staff increases or redeployment of staff to better advantage. Between 1966 and 1970 the numbers in receipt of weekly allowances rose by about half a million to more than two and a half million.

The number of claims during the course of a year rose from 3,800,000 in 1966 to over six million in 1970. Lump sum payments for exceptional needs rose from 372,000 to 560,000 and single immediate payments from about two and a half million to three and a half million. Although there were substantial staff increases during that period the inevitable time lag between the need and the increase in establishment meant that the period under consideration was one of considerable strain on local office staff, above all in relation to the sharp and unforeseen increase in numbers of callers, indicated by the steep rise in 'immediate payments'. The introduction in 1971 of the Family Income Supplement placed a further burden on Supplementary Benefits staff.

The SBC is an organisation set up to meet financial need promptly. The public is entitled to expect this and the pressure of social workers on behalf of a vulnerable and frequently inarticulate section of the community is much needed. Because the service is a financial one, however, the need is sometimes demonstrably urgent and is nearly always one which rouses feelings of urgency, both in claimant and in social worker, whatever the actual degree of that urgency. It is also easy to spot the mistakes. Perhaps social workers are fortunate in escaping such scrutiny; their delays and their inefficiencies are less in the public eye and arouse less emotion, except in those relatively few life and death situations, such as child neglect.

Whatever procedural improvements are made, the SBC will be left with the problem of individual motivation for the work; the degree of concern for individual claimants will affect technical and procedural efficiency. For example, procedural changes that diminish the continuity of concern for individual claimants may increase mistakes in calculations of entitlement. Those who seek to streamline organisation need to recognise the human factors in the quality of the service offered.

Judgement and Discretion

Are difficulties experienced by social workers in relation to those aspects of the Commission's powers that involve the exercise of judgement and discretion?

This has been discussed extensively in Chapter 2 as one of the most complex and important issues in relations between the SBC and social workers. There is no doubt that in the here and now this is a major area of difficulty for social workers. It is, of course, bound up with the general ignorance of the Supplementary Benefits scheme to which reference has been made earlier, and the publication of the Supplementary Benefits Handbook will go some way at least towards clarifying what is *not* discretionary and to giving some broad indications of discretionary powers. Most of the social workers to whom we spoke (contrary to the impression given by some pressure groups) readily took the point that discretion made public is no longer discretion. But they insisted that local variations in the exercise of discretion were confusing and inequitable. It seems there may need to be some further clarification between social workers and Supplementary Benefits staff of broad areas of discretion such as has been attempted in a recent document, 'Assistance in Cash', circulated to Directors of Social Service. In any case there are likely to be areas of local policy-making, somewhere between decisions on individual cases and policy requiring regional or Headquarters intervention. These will occur when local conditions (as for example large scale rehousing projects) create particular local problems. This can be negotiated at senior level between Managers and the heads of social work departments. The latter have sometimes been slow to seek clarification of policy on certain issues as, for example, in supplying furniture or paying removal expenses. What has happened is that the field workers—often young and/or inexperienced—have made an approach to an Executive Officer—sometimes equally young and/or inexperienced—on a specific case without the benefit of any formal guidance, past experience and accumulated mythology hanging like a cloud over the encounter.

Case Examples

The following three case examples must be given in minute detail if they are to illustrate the day-to-day problems of relationship that arise. Many of the issues they raise have in fact been discussed earlier in this book. Others cannot be pursued here. They are given at this point to bring to life the situations any social worker and any Executive Officer can expect to encounter and in which they will be expected to cooperate. They exemplify two of the knottiest problems in relationships between the two—unemployed men and the cohabitation rule.

Case Example A

Claimant: Mr George
Social Worker: Mr Montague (Senior Mental Welfare Officer)
This case was submitted by the Area Office as illustrating a lack of action by the Mental Welfare Department in dealing with a claimant considered to be in need of psychiatric treatment.

The claimant was 43 years of age, single and of no fixed abode. He lived rough in local woods and normally slept 'under the stars' except during inclement weather when he sheltered under a piece of canvas. His last regular work was for three years up to July 1957 when he was employed by Boots Limited as a shop assistant. His only other work since then was for two months in 1958, again as a shop assistant. In 1959 his unemployment benefit was exhausted and he has been in continuous receipt of assistance and supplementary benefit since. Over the years the local office has made strenuous efforts to get this man back into the employment field. He has convictions, mostly for larceny, although in 1959 he received a five months sentence for assaulting the police and the Clerk to the Magistrates' Court. When last convicted in 1967 he was bound over for a year.

In their efforts to obtain work for this claimant the staff at the local office arranged for him to attend a local advisory sub-committee meeting, and he was offered vacancies at an Industrial Rehabilitation Unit and a Re-establishment Centre, both of which he declined to accept. Although the local office staff reported at an early stage that the claimant was rather 'strange' the first reference to any mental condition was in October 1963 when a visiting officer reported: 'It may be his mental state, he draws his lips back like a mad dog when being questioned'. In May 1964 a confidential report of a hospital psychiatrist came into the possession of the local Manager via a member of the Discharged Prisoner's Aid Society who was trying to help the claimant find work. This stated that he was a paranoic and pointed out that there was no known cure for this condition although it was possible to control the most difficult symptoms. The report went on to state that he had been dealt with under Section 72 of the Mental Health Act and removed to a psychiatric hospital in 1960. Here he was uncooperative and refused all treatment until finally escaping. As a result of this information the local office referred the case to Headquarters for guidance and after further correspondence it was decided to approach the Local Authority Mental Welfare Officer for his guidance. In turn he consulted the Consultant Psychiatrist who was of the opinion that there were no grounds for the man's compulsory admission to hospital and it was pointed out that, when previously undergoing psychiatric hospital treatment, he refused all medication and would not take part in any therapeutic activities. It was finally arranged for the Special Welfare Officer to interview the claimant which she did but without success. In the end—in November 1966—with Headquarters' agreement he was deemed unemployable and registration at the local

Employment Exchange was waived, payment being made by order book. The situation has continued unchanged ever since.

The case was first discussed with the Deputy Manager who had a good knowledge of it. He strongly criticised the Mental Welfare Department for their lack of action. He accepted that the claimant had some form of mental condition but felt that it was the duty of the Mental Welfare Officer to constantly be in touch with him to try and persuade him to take treatment—the object being to get him to return to employment. It was also felt that the Mental Welfare Department had a duty to keep an eye on the claimant in view of the conditions he was living under. As it was, nothing was currently being done, no attempt was being made to keep in contact and he had been 'written off at forty-three'. There appeared to be no long-term plan of action and eventually the claimant would 'die in the woods'. Social workers were always referring to the casework they did yet here was a case crying out for action as far as the local office staff were concerned, and yet the social work agency concerned was inactive. As far as the Deputy Manager was concerned this case illustrated that the Mental Welfare Department 'did not wish to know' when a difficult case arose.

The case was then discussed with Mr Montague, Senior Mental Welfare Officer, who has had dealings with Mr George over many years. His approach to the case was quite clear and was summed up in a few words. The claimant was hostile and uncooperative to authority. Everything had been tried without success at all. He had been in prison and in psychiatric hospitals without improving his condition in any way. It was quite useless to try and persuade him to take any form of treatment. Further spells in either a mental hospital or prison would have ne effect. Section 30 action by the Department would also be ineffective. The case was considered to be a hopeless one and as long as the claimant's conduct did not seriously interfere with others he could live in whatever manner he chose. There was nothing that could be done within the terms of the Mental Health Act on a compulsory basis. There was the paradox that if he was willing to co-operate with the Mental Welfare Department he would not be the problem he is at present.

It is relatively easy to see in this case that the local office were unrealistic in their approach to Mr George's employment prospects. Their criticisms of the Mental Welfare Officers were not, however, simply on these grounds but because Mr George appeared to have been written off so far as any form of hospital or community care was concerned. This is just the kind of issue in which proper discussion between the parties could help each to appreciate the others' point of view. It may be that a man such as Mr George is indeed unhelpable in the present state of knowledge and resources. Equally he may not have been well handled by the social workers although in this case it is difficult to see that more could have been done. But the example serves to show the feeling which can build up.

Case Example B

Claimant: Mrs Horne
Social Worker: Mr Wilkins (Social Worker, Children's Department)

Mrs Horne, aged 38 years, divorced 1966, three children at school. In receipt of NA/SB for a number of years until July 1968 when supplementary benefit was withdrawn following a suspicion of cohabitation. This case illustrates contact between a social worker and a local office; there was a difference of opinion over the circumstances in which supplementary benefit had been withdrawn.

The social worker had first become involved in the case in February 1969 after the local NSPCC Inspector had reported that the children were being left alone at night because Mrs Horne was going out with a man called Bert Law. Mrs Horne was a woman of low mentality, divorced from her husband. A maintenance order of £6 a week had never been paid. She had taken no action to enforce payment because her ex-husband had threatened to assault her if she did so. He also found that Mr Law was calling on Mrs Horne two or three times a week and taking her out. He formed the opinion that Mr Law was a married man who was taking advantage of Mrs Horne's low mentality. The question of possible cohabitation did not arise in his mind at that time.

During February to early summer another case-worker visited Mrs Horne about twice a month. In July he went on holiday and when he returned he found that the supplementary benefit had been withdrawn and that, because of this, Mrs Horne had abandoned the children and they had been taken into care. It is fair to add, however, that her inadequate care of them was already a source of concern and they might have been taken into care anyway. Mr Wilkins, the social worker, thereupon telephoned the local office and was told that supplementary benefit had been withdrawn because (a) she was cohabiting with Mr Law and (b) her former husband should be supporting her. He went to see Mrs Horne but she was difficult and he could get nowhere with her on this occasion. He spoke to the local office who said Mr Horne should be supporting his ex-wife but that another officer was dealing with the case. He spoke to that officer who said the case had been on special investigation and that he had no hesitation in keeping supplementary benefit withdrawn especially now the children were in care; neighbours had said that Law was in the house in the evenings. The officer wondered in any case whether Mrs Horne was a suitable mother. (Mr Wilkins himself did not quite know what Mrs Horne was like as a mother. He said that there were poor material conditions in the home but that emotional conditions were better and should take priority in forming any judgement.)

When Mr Wilkins saw Mrs Horne next (at another address) he found that her only income was family allowance (18s) which she should not have been drawing in any case (with children in care) but decided to do nothing about this. Rent arrears were also building up. He again spoke to the local officer and told him what he had found and also why Mrs Horne would not take enforcement action against her ex-husband. The officer countered by saying that Mr Law should support Mrs Horne and he would not go into details because the matter was confidential. Mr Wilkins was quite clear in his mind that there was no regular cohabitation: he added that there seemed to be great difficulty in getting agreement on the definition of cohabitation. Because he was not satisfied with the position he consulted the Children's Officer who decided to take the case to a higher level and so she telephoned the Deputy Manager who said that he would have to read the reports. When Mr Wilkins telephoned again and spoke to the Manager, he thought supplementary benefit should not be paid but added that he would reconsider the case and offered to send a visitor to see Mrs Horne. Mr Wilkins said he would be willing to support an appeal if it were made.

Two days later the Department Manager telephoned Mr Wilkins and said that a visit had been made to Mrs Horne: she was not at home but a statement had been taken from a neighbour who said that Mr Law and Mrs Horne had gone away again and that the local office were reasonably satisfied that Mrs Horne was cohabiting. Mr Wilkins now began to wonder whether the local office might be right. The Court case in fact was adjourned twice and at the third hearing Mr Wilkins suggested that the children would be better in care in view of the circumstances: they were now less dependent on their mother who could give only a limited standard of care and they seemed to be happy in the Children's Home. As to Mrs Horne she found a job as a cleaner;

the Housing Department took over her former house and promised to re-house Mrs Horne if the children ever came home.

Examination of the case-paper showed that the local office staff knew that Mrs Horne was 'mentally slow'. The High Court order of £6 had been assigned to the local office but never paid. She had been interviewed in July 1969 by the LRO about this to see if she would seek enforcement of the order. She said she did not wish to do this, had decided to live with her boyfriend, and surrendered her order book. (The ex-husband had made it obvious he had persuaded her to do this to avoid action against him.) However, a week later Mr Law wrote to the local office to say he was not living with Mrs Horne and that he lived with his parents about fourteen miles away. The LRO noted in the case-paper that until it had been established where Mr Law lived it must be assumed that he lived with Mrs Horne. The latter called at the office two days later to say the children had been taken into care for twenty-eight days and that she was starting work in two weeks. No grant was made. A week later Mr Law called with Mrs Horne to deny cohabitation but refused to give his address. No grant was made to Mrs Horne.

The children may be 'better off in a home' but it is not hard to imagine similar situations in which this would not be so and in which grave harm could have been done to a woman and to her children through the withdrawal of an allowance in these circumstances. Mrs Horne's low mentality and poor care of the children are all too familiar complications of a situation in which external events can tip the balance of family stability up or down.

Case Example C

The following example is of a different kind. Here we have a woman of better intelligence and a situation in which there seems little doubt that she was cohabiting. It is included as an example of what might be described as 'mutual non-cooperation'. But the essential issue is that the muddle of all concerned placed Mrs Irons in an impossible situation.

Claimant: Mrs Irons

EO: Miss Rolph

Social Worker: Mrs Board (Children's Department)

The Children's Department believed that their efforts to establish the family after the children's discharge from care were hampered by the local office's objections to cohabitation. Mrs Irons' five children had been taken into care following the break-up of her marriage which resulted in divorce in January 1967. She came to Birmingham, where she lived in furnished rooms, and worked as a waitress. During this period she claimed supplementary benefit two or three times because of temporary illnesses.

In February 1967 she moved into a local authority house and the Children's Department became involved in bringing the children out of care and settling them with their mother. At the beginning of April 1967, Mrs Irons ceased work and the children were returned to her. She claimed supplementary benefit and was visited by the EO. Mrs Irons was 30, and her children were aged 12, 10, 8, 6 and 4. There was a court order of £6 a week against her ex-husband for the maintenance of the children but he had never paid it. He had remarried and had another family. Mrs Irons volunteered the information that she had a boyfriend whom she hoped to marry, but stressed that they were not living together. The EO decided to pay the allowance on a weekly basis pending liable relative action.

When Mrs Irons next called at the office to collect her money she took a Mr Coles, with her—whom she admitted had been living with her. When they were told that she could not receive supplementary benefit while he was living with her he said he would leave at once. The EO visited the next day to discuss the situation. Mrs Irons said he had left, and she did not know where he was. However there was a man in the house (and a car outside) but the man was said to be a carpenter come to mend the cupboards. The EO warned Mrs Irons that she could be prosecuted for making false statements. On return to the office Miss Rolph confirmed with the counter EO, who had seen Mrs Irons, that the man she had seen in the house looked like Mr Coles. She also found out that the car was registered in his name. She went to see Mrs Irons again the next day. There was delay in answering the door. Mrs Irons told her she should be more concerned about the welfare of the children than checking upon Mr Coles who was no concern of hers. Mrs Irons continued to deny that Mr Coles was still living with her, although it was fairly clear that he was hiding in the garden (Mrs Irons took Miss Rolph all over the house but would not open the door into the garden). His car was parked in the street and his clothes were in Mrs Irons' bedroom. Also on the same day it was confirmed with another area office that Mr Coles' wife and children were living on supplementary benefit, and that a court order had been made against him for £11 10s a week, but that he had said he was sick and unemployed. It was decided that nothing could be done except to pay Mrs Irons (she received her full allowance for the next two weeks), and submit the case for special investigation.

The Special Investigator observed the house and saw Mr Coles leave it early in the morning to go to work. He then interviewed Mrs Irons at length. She admitted that Mr Coles had lived with her in the past and that when he became sick and wanted to claim sickness benefit she had prevented him from doing so because she thought notice of his claim would be brought to the attention of the Supplementary Benefits office and, therefore, she had taken him with her to the office to explain the position and to get it sorted out. She denied that Mr Coles was living with her at present but she did not know where he lived although he called each morning and evening. The Special Investigator explained to her that (a) if Mr Coles lived with and kept her and her children he could apply for the court order in respect of his wife to be varied, and (b) she could enforce the maintenance order against her ex-husband. She said she wished she had been told this in the first place, that she would discuss it with Mr Coles, and intimated that she would probably no longer require supplementary benefit. The Special Investigator told her that if she did require further supplementary benefit she would be required to say where Mr Coles was living. He instructed the local office that if she did re-claim a maximum payment of £2 should be made until Mr Coles' address could be verified.

Mrs Irons called at the office in May 1967 to make a further claim and gave Mr Coles' address as her sister's house. She was paid £6 10s pending investigation. A visit was paid to the sister who confirmed that Mr Coles was living there, although there was considerable doubt about this (the sister was warned about 'aiding and abetting'). Mrs Irons called at the Area Office again on 9 May and 16 May and each time was paid £12—'related to normal earnings figure in view of known circumstances' and 'pending TEO decision'. When she called on 9 May Mrs Irons said she had been to court about the court order against her husband. The LRO telephoned the Probation Officer on 10 May. He said both Mrs Irons and Mr Coles had been to see him and that he had advised Mr Coles not to continue living with Mrs Irons at present as he could not keep her (he said he earned £18 a week and his commitments, with the Court order for his wife and children, were £26 a week), and because he prejudiced her claim to supplementary benefit. It was accepted that Mr Coles must have left the house and as Mrs Irons said she hoped to return to work anyway, an order book was issued for the full amount of supplementary benefit from 20 May 1968.

Mrs Irons was visited again by the EO in June 1968 and was said to be 'extremely cooperative and very pleasant'. She said she would be returning to work and would make arrangements with a neighbour to look after the children when they were not at school. She returned to work as a waitress at the beginning of July.

Discussion with the social workers showed that there was in fact no disagreement as to whether Mrs Irons was in fact cohabiting and it was clear that this fact was known to the social workers when they were visiting. The social worker felt, however, that the rule as it stood placed the couple in an impossible position.

It must be pointed out however, that the full implications of this situation had not been adequately considered by either side. Both seemed more concerned with their agency role, as they saw it, than with the realities of Mrs Irons' situation. The Supplementary Benefits officer seemed concerned only with the point that supplementary benefit could not be paid to a woman who was cohabiting, and the social worker only with the question of the children remaining at home regardless of the financial implications. There is little doubt that Mrs Irons and Mr Coles were living together as man and wife all the time, perhaps from before Mrs Irons moved to the new house. If this were so it raises the following points:

(a) In bringing the children out of care the social worker should have taken account of the fact that the mother was cohabiting and what this would mean in financial terms, in view of the legal position. It seemed that the social workers involved had thought of cohabitation as nothing much to do with them.

(b) Nobody, except the Special Investigating Officer, seems to have considered all the financial implications of this case. So far as known the situation was that Mrs Irons had five children for whom there was a court order of £6 against her ex-husband. The court order had not been paid to Mrs Irons, and it is not known whether the father maintained the children while they were in care. Whether or not the father could be made to pay the order was a very material consideration, but the Children's Department did not appear to have given any thought to this, and the SBC had been slow in following it up, so that it had never been resolved. It seems, in fact, that the father, as he had married again and has another family, was unable to pay the order.

(c) Mr Coles, the cohabitee, had a court order of £11 10s to pay for his wife and children. Neither the Supplementary Benefits official nor the social worker found out whether Mr Coles paid the order or not.

(*d*) Mrs Irons and Mr Coles, in setting up a home together were placed in an impossible financial situation—if she were not to receive the court order for her children and he had to pay the order for his wife and children. The situation could have been resolved if it had been accepted that they were living as man and wife, Mr Irons had applied for a variation in his Court order and a supplementary benefit allowance had been made for the children whilst the Court order for them was not being paid. Only the Special Investigating Officer ever began to approach the case in this way. At no time was there any contact between the two about the matter, and it seemed that to the Children's Department any contact would have been regarded as an embarrassment. It is no wonder that Mrs Irons was devious. Bringing her children out of care and setting her up in a new house placed her, in the light of her relationship with Mr Coles, in an intolerable situation in which she had knowingly to make fraudulent statements to this Department. Both Mrs Board and Miss Rolph said she was a good mother and good manager. She solved the dilemma herself, to some extent, by returning to work despite having five children to care for. A depressing story.

The evidence is overwhelming that there is much room for improvement in the relationships between social work and Supplementary Benefits staff. Some improvement in relationships can only occur when each puts its own house in order, in terms of organisation, procedure, training and so on. Some difficulties, as analysed in the earlier part of this book, appear intractible without radical and far-reaching changes in the present system and will continue to give rise to tensions in the relationships between the two. To some extent—but not, in the opinion of the writer, to the present extent—tensions may be needed to preserve a balance between conflicting interests in society. The very word 'tension', however, is in itself hopeful, implying as it does some connection between objects. One of the most depressing aspects of the writer's period as Social Work Adviser was not the discovery of tension but of apathy, indifference and misconceived hostility based upon mutual ignorance.

Implications for Social Work Education
This has, therefore, important implications for the education and

training of social workers and Supplementary Benefits staff. The training of the latter has already been considered and it is clearly important that it should include as much instruction about, and contact with, social workers as is possible in a very short period with many other competing priorities. However, it is upon social workers whose professional education is anything between four and eight times as long as the inservice training of an Executive Officer that the main responsibility for such learning should rest. This is a period when attitudes are formed, when interest is aroused and when the would-be social worker is free to absorb knowledge. Until recently, the majority of social work students have only encountered the SBC through their work with particular clients. They have had a client's eye-view— often salutary and distressing—but have had little opportunity to understand some of the complexities involved in the scheme and the roles and functions of the Supplementary Benefits official. In this, there is no doubt that the SBC has been tardy. Suggestions, for example, of student placements within Supplementary Benefits offices seemed at first to raise insuperable administrative difficulties of the kind which made the sceptic detect ambivalence. However, limited experiments[1] are now under way and insignificant as they are numerically, they represent a major advance. Their success and expansion will depend almost entirely on the way students and educators use them. If they are seen as an opportunity 'to put spies on the camp' (and no doubt some Supplementary Benefits officials will fear this) the experiments may founder, in which case it may well be that the scene will be set for intractible and institutionalised conflict between social work and income maintenance services. As a professional, the student should be concerned first to understand the problems he sees. Only thus can he evolve an appropriate strategy—whether of mediation or confrontation at local or at national levels. This book has been written in the hope of providing some of the background knowledge the social worker needs to understand what he sees. But the addition of live, personal experience for students is essential. The present trends in social work, with increased awareness of the importance of the broad spectrum of social services in the lives of clients, brings with it the responsibility to apply rational and objective understanding to those services.

The Social Work Element within the SBC

It is doubtful, however, whether more than limited progress can be made without the introduction into the Supplementary Benefits scheme

[1] Small groups of social work students have had short placements in local offices.

of a 'social work element' and a more precise definition at local office level of responsibility for liaison with social workers. The former has been approved in principle by the Commission, as witnessed by the appointment of a Social Work Adviser and the intention to appoint Regional Social Work Service Officers. Their role will be to contribute towards liaison with social workers in outside agencies; to assist with certain aspects of training; and with cases of special difficulty involving social or psychological difficulties. It would be naive to suppose that their appointment will be warmly welcomed throughout the SBC, given the suspicion of professionals and the doubtful status of social workers. In the light of the discussions in earlier chapters, it is easy to see how valuable a contribution they might make but equally easy to see that their impact may depend in the first instance—as with all social workers in secondary settings—as much on individual skill as on the accepted authority of professional expertise.

Local Office Liaison with Social Workers

Local office organisation in relation to welfare and to liaison with social workers needs also to be considered. Local offices vary greatly in the priority they accord to this aspect of their work and they organise it differently. The majority regard such referral and liaison as the responsibility of the Territorial Executive Office in whose area the claimant lives; the Manager or Deputy Manager is a last resort in cases of difficulty. This is strongly defended by senior officials on the grounds that it encourages the officer concerned to have proper regard for welfare and is an integral part of his task. It is, of course, essential that the TEO and visiting CO should watch out for any need for welfare services. It is argued that, were these functions taken away from the TEO, it would lead to a diminution of concern for these aspects of claimants' well-being. Given sufficient emphasis by management and in training, in particular in the improved systems of referral discussed earlier, it would seem that such arrangements could work well in the majority of cases for which referral and liaison are relatively straightforward. Difficulties arise, however, in the minority of complex cases with which much of this book has been concerned. In such circumstances it would seem to be much more satisfactory if formal liaison were established with a particular official designated as having responsibility for these matters. It is open to argument whether such liaison should include responsibility for working with the minority of difficult cases. Probably it should since an intervening 'liaison officer' might lead to further complications in communication. The arguments

P

for such a post are fourfold: first, these cases are always time-consuming. The job of the Executive Officer is not structured so as to permit the kind of discussion that may be necessary. Secondly, Executive Officers vary greatly in their interest in their side of the work. It is unfair to expect them to show an equal degree of concern for a social worker's clients and equally unfair that clients should be affected by the prejudice or indifference of some. Thirdly, a local office specialist would convey to the rest of the staff the importance the Commission attaches to this part of the work. Fourthly, social workers, building up confidence in a named and known person, would find the approach to Supplementary Benefits offices easier and would in time learn more of its workings than by the present intermittent contact with frequently changing staff. Such a liaison officer must, of course, take care not to usurp the role of the social worker. Indeed it might be part of his function to bring more effective pressure to bear on social work agencies than the average Executive Officer has time or inclination for. The new social service departments of local authorities also offer the possibility of regular contact with such an officer who might, for example, visit departments to deal with inquiries or even work with social workers in family advice centres, as they develop.

Social Workers' Organisational Responsibility

So far, this has been a one-sided discussion of ways in which the SBC might, through its own internal organisation, relate to social workers more effectively. What of the social workers? Exactly the same arguments apply to social work 'specialists' in relation to social security as have been given in reverse. Certainly, to divorce this aspect of clients' welfare from the social and psychological problems with which the ordinary social worker must deal would be retrogressive in the light of present trends. On the other hand the field social worker needs expert advice and, on occasion, support in contacts with Supplementary Benefits over individual cases. There seems a strong case for specialist appointments to this end which would have particular relevance to the issue of discretionary powers discussed earlier.[1] But the success of such arrangements turns in the end on a degree of mutual confidence and a willingness to negotiate even when conflict is strong.

For Supplementary Benefits officials, practical measures will convince more effectively than instructions that their seniors care about this side of their work. As has been shown, this has been evident in a

[1] This was attempted by the Children's Department of one local authority.

variety of ways, of which the most important are probably the development of specialist training and the appointments—present and pending
—of social work officers. Unfortunately, however, the impact of these
and other developments is slow to reach local offices. There has been
uncertainty in the minds of many officers as to how much value their
seniors will place on the kind of activity involved in referral and
liaison. This is in part a problem of communication which so frequently
exists between Headquarters and local levels in any organisation. It
also stems in part from a fundamental conflict of interests within
Headquarters between protection of public funds and concern for
welfare of individuals. But to understand the present situation social
workers must grasp the differences between the professional and the
bureaucratic orientation. Despite the scepticism of some individuals,
the Supplementary Benefits official will, by virtue of his role, usually do
as he is told. His position is intolerable if he is subjected to too great a
degree of role conflict or (as is now sometimes the case) when he
does not know what he is being told to do. But by and large he is not
uneasy within his structure if his instructions are clear and his task
defined. If one adds to this the fact that the majority of officials are, as
individuals, humane and concerned about their claimants, if bewil-
dered by their vagaries, and that attempts are being made in training to
provide them with greater understanding of claimants, the situation
need not be seen as desperate. But there are may unknowns of which,
as has been suggested earlier, the impact of training as it is provided
within this administrative framework is probably the most significant.

So far as the social workers are concerned, the writer is convinced
that for the majority, greater knowledge of the Supplementary Benefits
scheme and organisation is bound to lead to improvements in relationships; not because criticism will thus be deflected—in fact it may be
increased—but because it will ensure that the criticism is better
directed and better informed. It may also on occasions enable credit to
be given where it is due.

This book has been written on the basis of the assumption that
social workers do want to know more about the Supplementary
Benefits Commission and that they need, not a scapegoat, but a partner
with whom they can at times be angry and at times content. Much will
depend on the direction the profession takes in the next ten years and
on whether, in incorporating the initiatives concerned with greater
social and political involvement, social work can preserve some of the
self-and-other awareness which was its earlier emphasis.

P*

UNEMPLOYMENT RESEARCH

(M. Hill)

In a situation of reasonably full employment it is popularly believed that the long-term or frequently unemployed can be divided into two categories: those who have disabilities that affect their ability to get or keep work; and those who are not effectively trying to get work. The shorthand expressions used for extreme cases in these two categories are the 'unemployables' and the 'workshy'. Our research task would be easy if these two discrete categories of popular mythology were readily identifiable, but of course low employability and low motivation to work are often interrelated. Furthermore both these phenomena are significantly affected by the strength of the demand for labour, not just in general terms but in relation to different areas and skills. Our task, therefore, is: (a) to examine what proportion of the long-term or frequently unemployed are in fact distinguished by characteristics that set them clearly apart from those who move off the unemployed registers fairly easily; (b) to study the complex interaction of factors that play a part in the unemployment problems of those whose difficulties are not so readily explained by simple characteristics, developing a system of typologies to organise this task; and (c) to attempt to frame some indices that will add up to a balance of probabilities that a man will have difficulties in obtaining employment.

In undertaking a task of this kind our main difficulty lies in getting behind the major factors which repeated studies have identified as being correlated with long-term unemployment—age, poor health and low skill in particular—to develop a more sophisticated causal analysis of the problem. For example, men over fifty with severe disabilities and little skill who fall out of work do not always remain unemployed until they retire. Is it just chance that distinguishes those in this category who get work from those who remain unemployed or are these social and psychological factors that help to explain the differential job-seeking success of men in very similar general categories? We are naturally concentrating our attention on men in lower risk categories than those in the above example but it demonstrates the nature of the explanatory dilemmas we face.

Three areas have been selected for the research; Newcastle upon Tyne, Coventry, and the London Borough of Hammersmith. The latter two areas had, at the time the research was planned, unemployment well below the national average. Newcastle was included to provide a contrasting area of above average unemployment. However, during the months immediately prior to going into the field, unemployment rose dramatically in Coventry. So the final situation is that we are comparing three areas, one with continuing low unemployment, one with persistent high unemployment, and one with current high unemployment but a history of low unemployment. Nevertheless in all three areas it is still the case that a high proportion of those who fall out of work get new jobs in under three months so it is still valid to try to sort out the factors that distinguish the 'stickers' from the short-term unemployed.

We have avoided the adoption of any arbitrary definition of long-term or frequent unemployment. Our sample is a proportion (one-tenth in Newcastle and Coventry, one-fifth in Hammersmith) of all the men on the Department of Employment unemployment registers on 1 October 1971. It therefore includes men who have or will have (we have a six month follow-up period) spells of unemployment of all durations from one day to six months or more. These men are given an interview dealing with their family and domestic backgrounds, health, education, work experience and attitudes to work. Information on their employment histories and on their sickness records are acquired from the Department of Employment and the Department of Health and Social Security, and on their criminal records (if any) from the Home Office. All these factors can then be related to their experience of unemployment. Subsequently, in one of the three areas, Coventry, a sub-sample of low-skilled and relatively young men with records of considerable unemployment over the past three years will be given a second interview that will probe their attitudes and situations in depth. These interviews will be conducted by trained social workers, and will provide qualitative material to put alongside the wide range of quantifiable material acquired in the initial interviews.

At the time of writing (November 1971) the field work on the first-stage interviews is nearing completion. The interviews of the sub-sample will be conducted early in 1972. Publications of a preliminary report (Cambridge University Press 'Men Out of Work') will be in the Spring of 1973. A further analysis will, it is hoped, appear in 1975.

ACTION RESEARCH

(A. R. Thompson)

The evaluation of the Supplementary Benefits Commission's work with the long-term and frequently unemployed represents one element of the research project commissioned at the University of Oxford under the direction of Miss Olive Stevenson by the Department of Health and Social Security. The Supplementary Benefits Handbook notes the Commission's procedures for the control of voluntary unemployment (paras 162–182) which include review of claimants selected on specified criteria by a specially trained group of officers. The process of review involves an assessment—on the basis of existing records and interviews—of the claimants' personal situation and its effect on his employment prospects and, in the light of this assessment, activity including referral to medical or social work agencies, specific help with finding employment, general encouragement, retraining, and in a few cases, prosecution. Underlying this activity is the Commission's responsibility to 'exercise its functions in such manner as shall best promote the welfare of persons affected by the exercise thereof'.

When we turn to this concept of welfare underlying the activity of the officer, problems of definition occur. Achieving the return to work of a man with a long record of unemployment may not of itself be a contribution to his welfare—the effect upon his family in emotional or even material terms may well counterbalance any benefits accruing to him from the simple fact of being in paid employment. The Commission's Unemployment Review Officers, in forming their assessment and casework plan, are required to take into consideration the total functioning of the individual and not necessarily to work towards his future employment as a total objective. An appropriate goal may not be employment, at least in the short term, and success may better be indicated by improvements effected in social, psychological, physical and material areas of the claimant's functioning which have represented serious obstacles to his employability. Similarly, welfare considerations must apply not only to objectives of the worker's activity, but to the activity itself. Although the claimants' entitlement to financial aid is subject to a behavioural condition, it would seem reasonable to see some limitation on the persuasive/coercive activity of the officer encompassed within the welfare requirement, but again only the most general guidelines, such as are afforded by law, are available. Indeed a more general question is raised concerning the attachment of a behavioural condition to the granting of material aid; may this in itself be contrary to the notion of welfare?

The existence of this control procedure suggests that a distinction may be made between the voluntarily unemployed—those exploiting the system in a rational way—and the involuntarily unemployed—those whose employability is limited by any of a variety of physical, psychological or social handicaps. The grosser forms of handicap are readily evident. There is, however, no clear-cut division between the employable and the unemployable, even among these cases, but rather employability is a product of a complex of environmental and individual factors. Similarly the distinction between handicapped and non-handicapped is not clear cut: social, psychological and physical factors and their interplay create a picture whose complexity is underestimated by any simple division.

The problems faced by Unemployment Review Officers, insofar as they are solvable at a fieldwork level, set a high value on skills of personal interaction; knowledge of psychological, physical and social determinants of the individual's behaviour and situation; of the extent to which these lend themselves to amelioration; and of the ameliorative techniques themselves. There exist specialists in the relevant disciplines to whom referral may be made, but the sifting process prior to referral is crucial and its effeciency might be expected to be determined by the level of skill and knowledge applied in it.

The present research project is seeking to clarify some of these issues which involve both the process and the results of unemployment review activity. It is planned to introduce some variation in activity which, apart from serving as a yardstick against which current practice may be measured, may also provide some useful indication of the direction which future policy may most appropriately take. The range of variation is limited by relevant law. It is, however, possible to introduce procedures which, at one extreme, are based on more fully developed skills and knowledge in social casework and social studies generally and, at the other extreme, reduce to a minimum the impact of the behavioural condition on the claimant.

The study, in its evaluation of social intervention, is concerned with cause and effect relationships. The design must afford control over the manipulation of stimuli and the assignment of subjects and therefore a formal experimental design, rather than a survey has been adopted. Four comparison groups are proposed, consisting of:

(a) claimants falling within the sample who would be subject to no special review action
(b) claimants allocated to normal review by Unemployment Review officers
(c) claimants allocated to review by UROs supported by social work consultants
(d) claimants allocated to review by professionally qualified social workers supported by social work consultants.

The experiment will last for one year and will take place in six areas throughout England. In each area claimants will be randomly allocated to each comparison group; a limited sample will be selected from each group and the cases of those so selected will be studied in some detail. A large amount of information will be readily available on the situation of the claimants, on the method of working of the officer (including frequency and content of officer-claimant contact, referrals and contacts with other agencies, etc.), and on the effects of that intervention on the employment record of the claimant. As well as seeking information of this sort, the project is concerned to give full weight to the notion of welfare and to seek indicators of the impact of the intervention that go beyond a simple count of work record. The claimant's own view of his situation and of his reaction to the review process will be sought in independent interviews and consideration is being given to objective measures of change in psychosocial functioning.

The research project may serve to clarify the effects and effectiveness of the existing practices of unemployment review and may provide empirical evidence relevant to future developments. In addition, it is envisaged that a contribution will be made to our knowledge of the process and product of social casework generally. The setting and focus of the activity to be studied is unusual in casework practice. It is, however, an area that demands skill and sensitivity in practice and has a very real impact on the material, social, and psychological well-being of the recipients of the service.

FURTHER READING ON
VOLUNTARY UNEMPLOYMENT

For examples of work that throws light on family interaction and that might profitably be related to the study of voluntary unemployment, see:

N. ACKERMAN, *The Psychodynamics of Family Life*, Basic Books Inc., New York, 1958.

K. BANNISTER and other, *Social Casework in Marital Problems*, Tavistock Publications, London, 1955.

R. D. LAING and A. ESTERSON, *Sanity, Madness, and the Family*, Tavistock Publications, London, 1969.

R. D. LAING, *Interventions in Social Situations*, Association of Family Caseworkers, 1969.

L. PINCUS and K. BANNISTER, *Shared Phantasy in Marital Problems*, Welwyn Codicote Press, 1965.

FURTHER READING ON
UNSUPPORTED MOTHERS

D. MARSDEN, *Mothers Alone: Poverty and the Fatherless Family*, Allen Lane, London, 1969.

P. MORRIS, *Prisoners and their Families*, Allen and Unwin, London, 1965.

M. WYNN, *Fatherless Families*, Michael Joseph, London, 1964.

In addition to published work, there are a number of research studies currently supported, or being undertaken, by the Department of Health and Social Security. These include:

(*a*) Study of the circumstances of one-parent families. (Offices of Population Censuses and Surveys)

(*b*) Study of separated wives receiving supplementary benefits. (SBC)

(*c*) Study of motherless families. (V. N. George, University of Nottingham.)

(*d*) Study of Adjustment to divorce. (R. L. C. Chester, University of Hull.)

(*e*) Study of unsupported mothers. (C. J. Picton, University of Leicester.)

(*f*) Comparative study of fatherless families and families of men who are chronically sick or unemployed. (SBC)